28 Days Weight Loss Plan

INSTANT FAT BURN SECRETS

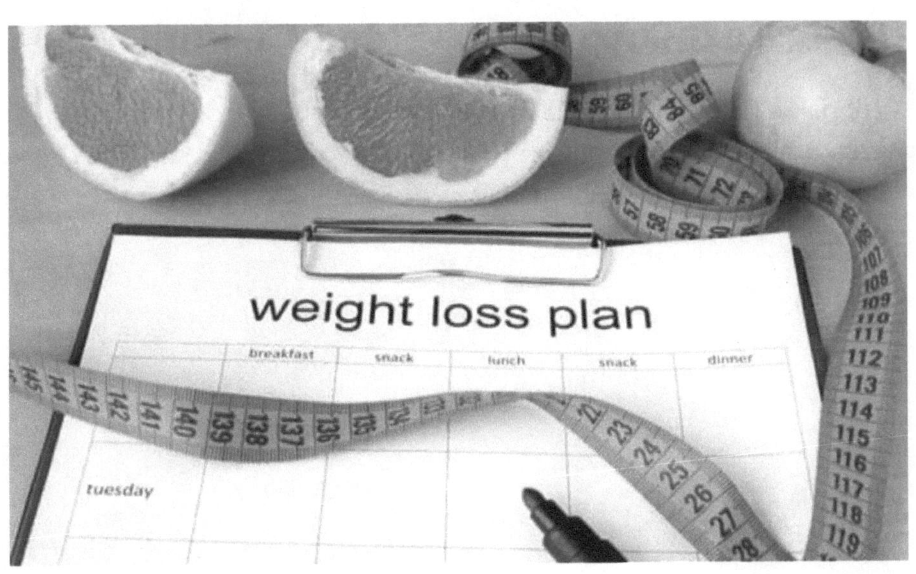

SIDNEY GRIFFITH

Legal & Disclaimer

The information contained in this book and its contents is not designed to replace or take the place of any form of medical or professional advice; and is not meant to replace the need for independent medical, financial, legal or other professional advice or services, as may be required. The content and information in this book has been provided for educational and entertainment purposes only.

The content and information contained in this book has been compiled from sources deemed reliable, and it is accurate to the best of the Author's knowledge, information and belief. However, the Author cannot guarantee its accuracy and validity and cannot be held liable for any errors and/or omissions. Further, changes are periodically made to this book as and when needed. Where appropriate and/or necessary, you must consult a professional (including but not limited to your doctor, attorney, financial advisor or such other professional advisor) before using any of the suggested remedies, techniques, or information in this book.

Upon using the contents and information contained in this book, you agree to hold harmless the Author from and against any damages, costs, and expenses, including any legal fees potentially resulting from the application of any of the information provided by this book. This disclaimer applies to any loss, damages or injury caused by the use and application, whether directly or indirectly, of any advice or information presented, whether for breach of contract, tort, negligence, personal injury, criminal intent, or under any other cause of action.

You agree to accept all risks of using the information presented inside this book.

You agree that by continuing to read this book, where appropriate and/or necessary, you shall consult a professional (including but not limited to your doctor, attorney, or financial advisor or such other advisor as needed) before using any of the suggested remedies, techniques, or information in this book

TABLE OF CONTENTS

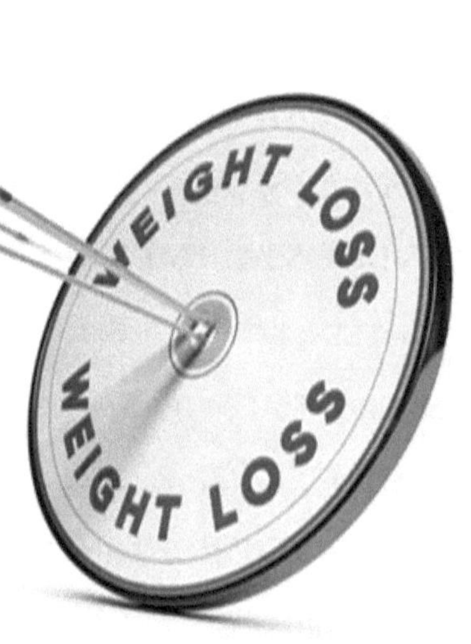

INTRODUCTION

If you're like the majority of people that are trying to lose weight, tone up and get fit, you've probably read countless weight loss books and tried all the fad diets. As you probably know by now those fad diets don't work, do they? And if you are one of the lucky ones to lose some weight while on the diet, how long do you manage to keep it off? As long as you stay on the diet right? As soon as you come off the diet you'll put it all back on, and then some.

And then there's the fat loss supplement industry, how many miracle pills have you popped? How many weight loss shakes have you already drank? When you fail on these as most people do you feel it's your fault, right? In reality it's not your fault.

Battling excess weight can be one of the most frustrating, challenging, and emotionally draining experiences on earth. Despite the numerous diets, exercise regimens, and magic pills for weight loss, Americans continue to grow larger and larger year after year. More than two thirds of the adult population and one third of our children are now overweight. Obesity rates have tripled since the 1960s.

I believe that most overweight people are actually naturally thin. The body is complex and designed to maintain healthiness. The body is smarter than any diet pill or fad diet on the market. If you just change your eating habits to align with your body's natural ability to heal, stay slim, and have energy, you will never have to worry about weight again.

The truth is that nobody wants to be fat. Excess weight is due to a combination of factors that are often outside of one's control, such as genetics, hormonal imbalances, or the poor quality Standard American Diet (SAD) readily available to us. It isn't your fault that you have problems with your weight. Even if you have enough willpower to keep yourself from eating when your brain tells you that you're hungry, you still may not be able to lose weight. There are so many other factors in play that cause you to gain weight. Until you understand the real reasons you gain weight, you will never be able to lose weight permanently. The key is to learn to naturally speed up your body's fat-burning capabilities to help you lose weight effortlessly and get healthy.

The good news is that anyone can lose weight and stay slim if he or she just understands, addresses, and corrects the hidden causes of weight gain. In order to succeed in the battle of the bulge, you have to realize that losing weight involves a major lifestyle change. In this ebook, I will share with you how to assist your own body in becoming naturally thin and healthy.

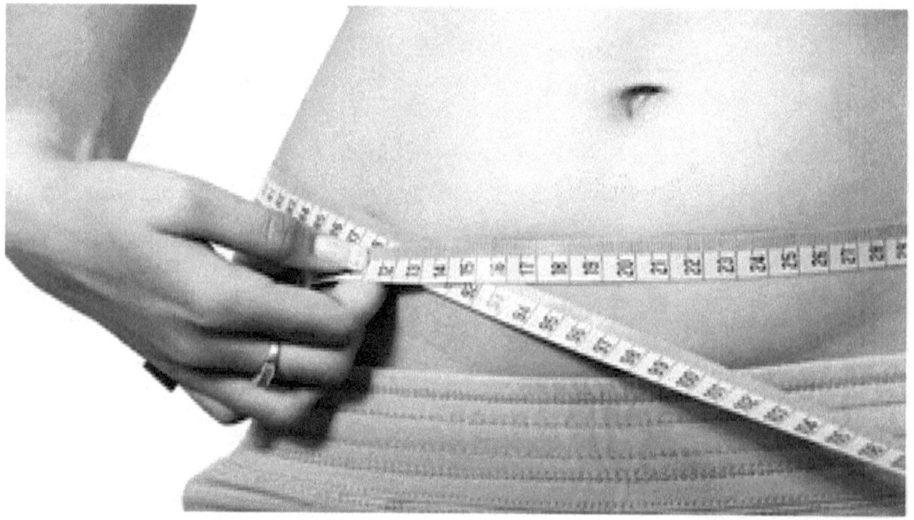

Chapter 1

Why You Can't Lose Weight

Six Reasons Why

Many people who are unsuccessful at controlling their body image will ask, **"Why can't I lose weight"**?

In this section, you will find seven reasons why most people have trouble burning calories, melting away fat and how to overcome those challenges.

1. You are consuming more calories than you burn.

You may be consuming more calories than you burn and that may even lead to weight gain. To correct this, make sure that you are consuming slightly less calories. Switching over from 3 square meals to 6 smaller ones may make it easier to consume fewer calories, just make sure that your meals are small enough to consume fewer calories. Weighing your food will also help you to get your portion sizes right.

2. You are burning fewer calories than you consume.

Your exercise might not be effective enough and you may be burning fewer calories than you consume. To counter this, all you have to do is to increase your exercise. If you want to lose weight, you have to exercise for at least 5 days a week - doing cardio and weight training. Making sure you move more and that you are more active will also help you to burn more calories.

3. Your exercise is ineffective for weight loss.

You may be doing exercise that is ineffective for weight loss - like light cardio and weight training. The best exercise for weight loss is cardio interval training, weight training (heavy weights) and any exercise that breaks you out in a sweat.

4. You craves junk food.

Hey, that's why we are overweight! Your body and brain has got used to it's sugar and junk food fix. But you will find if you stick at it the cravings will pass after a few weeks. When the cravings hit you make sure you always have some fruit with you to snack on. And use some willpower my friend!!

5. You forget about the little things you eat and the little bites you take.

You may forget about a bite here and a taste there - it can all make your weight loss difficult without even knowing it. To help you see where your eating are slipping up, keep a food dairy where you write everything down what you ate.

6. Relying on weight loss supplements

Most folks want to get rid of their body fat now so they turn to what they perceive as quick fix solutions. Taking expensive weight loss, pills will only drain your wallet. You may lose a few pounds here or there but you will not realize any long term benefit.

I hope this section has shed the light on the reasons why you can't lose weight and that you used this to correct the little mistakes that you where making so that you can start losing weight again.

Why our body craves certain food and should we listen to our cravings?

Sure, it's entirely normal to have food cravings. It's When you constantly give in to your cravings and overindulge, is when you pay the price, and notice a bulge occurring. Understand your cravings are part of life, you can take action to prevent giving in to them.

Everyone knows the formula for weight gain and weight loss:

Take in more calories than you burn = gain weight.

Burn more calories than you take in = weight loss.

Cravings from your body and brain tend to get in the way of our intended goals. To win the battle we need to know why cravings occur, and how to defeat them using healthy practices.

Why We Have Cravings?

There are many reasons people develop cravings throughout the day. Women tend to develop more cravings more often due to their wide range of hormonal swings, but men get cravings too... we just don't talk about it as much. 91% of women interviewed in a 2007 Tufts University study reported craving certain foods from time to time.

Familiar reasons for cravings:

Hormonal fluctuations.

Stress cause us to reach for comfort foods

Anxiety triggers desires as well as hormones

Nutritional deficiencies in the diet cause cravings for the missing

nutrients.

Low blood sugar caused by eating too infrequently.

Your body & brain are used to higher caloric

Specific trigger circumstances or feelings set off desire for certain foods.

Eating disorders.

Pregnancy multiplies the above factors.

Defeat Cravings

First you must understand your cravings. Assess your craving and determine if it is caused by a nutritional need or low in calories intake, or a certain vitamin or mineral. If you are not taking a quality multi-vitamin, this may be a great place to start.

Nutritional cravings are great because you can satisfy your craving while also helping your body at the same time. If you find yourself craving an unhealthy food, think about what nutrient that food contains that you may need. Example if you are craving ice cream, you may be deficient in calcium.

If you are craving a bag of potatoes chips you may need sodium, try eating a serving of lightly salted nuts, or a stick of beef jerky — Accept cravings as normal, but that does not mean you have to give in completely to them.

Those who maintain a healthy weight have learned how to manage their cravings by satisfying the basic need through moderation, and good solid nutritional supplementation. Keep in mind if you deny 100% of all your cravings there is a very high likelihood of disastrous binging.

What to do to repair and heal our body?

1. Eat Frequently

To manage your blood sugar, metabolism and appetite, schedule to eat 5-6 small meals or snacks every 2-3 hours throughout the day. Keep healthy snacks on hand at all times. **Some healthy snack ideas include:**

Fruit
Vegetables
Ginger & Green Tea
Nuts (Bake or Raw)
Whole Grain Crackers
Plant based seeds
Veggies Pickles

2. Drink water

Study after study proves you can keep your appetite at bay by drinking water all day long. Water itself can eliminate your cravings.

I recommend you look into the quality of the water you are drinking. Invest in a premium quality water filter system is essential since our body contain 70% water.

Avoid buying pre-packed water from the Supermarket, partly due to plastic waste and mostly is because the plastic bottle water may have contained tiny particles which is harmful to our body.

3. Delay your craving

When the craving hits you, you can set a goal and make that craving a reward for accomplishing your goal. (providing the craving is not for something totally unhealthy like chips or candy corn. "If I can resist my craving for 24 hours, I will reward myself with a small serving of ice cream."

Sometimes by delaying the craving, it will go away entirely, and you can skip the cheat altogether. If you do still want your craving, eat only a small portion. Understand before you even take your first bite that you are only going to have 3 bites, etc. if you are craving chocolate; just eat half the bar instead of the whole thing.

4. Snacking is not so bad

Most diet plans including doctor-directed weight loss plans say that snacking is, not always bad. You should be allowed 200-300 calories a day to eat whatever you want. This is not an invitation to suck down 50 grams of sugar all in one shot, but it should provide enough flexibility to eat that half bar of chocolate, one slice of pizza, a small bag of salted cashews, or whatever it is that you are craving.

Snacking is even better if it is food on the metabolism-boosting food list, things like an apple, broccoli, carrots, celery, and walnuts.

5. Supplement with high quality vitamins, minerals, and antioxidants

This will keep your body from randomly craving certain nutrients that can sometimes be found in foods that are not good for you.

Vitamins and minerals: I recommend you do not purchase your vitamins from any of the big box stores or pharmacies. Most of those big name brands may be cheap in price but believe me they are worth much less than you pay for them. Formulas for men and women are different. Different needs for different folks.

Antioxidants: I recommend everyone take antioxidants. The world in which we live, the food we eat and the air we breathe, enhances our bodies production of free radicals — a good quality antioxidant formulation is essential. Vitamin A, E, C are great antioxidants.

6. Use willpower and self talk to defeat the craving

When it comes down to the final straw, you need to show your toughness. If you find yourself craving sweets and you see a big piece of your favourite pie, just say no. The idea is to control your cravings and not let them control you — Listen to your body and work to understand why you are experiencing cravings.

Tell yourself every day, out loud that you are winning; you are losing weight, and inches.

Setting Reasonable Long Term Goals

People want to loss their weight for various reasons. Some people loss weight just to be healthier. Some others do it to look better and feel better. No matter what is the reason, the sensible and realistic goal is essential for successful weight loss and weight management. In order to succeed at weight loss, one must never under-estimate the power of effective goal-setting.

The most effective goal-setting system by far, is the **SMART** system.

SMART stands for:

Specific
Measurable
Action-Oriented
Realistic
Timed

You have a much greater change of reaching your weight loss goals, if you take some time take some time to conduct a SMART inventory - preferably in writing. **Here's how it's done:**

Step 1: SPECIFIC

You must make sure that the weight loss goals you set are as specific as possible.

A general/ambiguous goal would be: "I want to lose weight."

A specific goal would be: "I want to lose 10 pounds of fat by the end of February."

The former is a vague statement; such statements hold no credibility whatsoever, and do not have a sound psychological effect on your brain, whereas a specific goal has a much greater chance of accomplishment -- simply because it's stated in a non-ambiguous manner, hence - your brain registers it as an active goal (as opposed to passive, irrelevant grousing).

Make sure all the goals you set / statements you make are as specific as can be. You should apply this to everything, including your actual weight loss strategy. That is, instead of saying "I will eat less", you should establish how much you're going to eat, exactly. "Less" is not an action-oriented term -- at least your brain does not interpret it as such.

Step 2: MEASURABLE

Establish the HOW and the WHEN.

HOW are you going to measure your weight progress? Choose a method (or a combination of methods) that is suitable for you. It can be the scale, the measuring tape, your BMI, your body fat %, your hip-to-waist ration, clothing sizes, the mirror, or anything else you want to use.

Decide **WHEN** you're going to measure your weight loss progress. Every day (bad idea, by the way) ... every week... every fortnight?

Now, how will you know when you've accomplished your goal? Proceed with the end result in mind. What is your ultimate goal? Do you want to be able to fit into a particular dress (what size is it)? Do you want to see a particular number on the scale? Do you want to lose x inches off your waist?

It's a good idea to document your progress regularly.

Step 3: ACTION-ORIENTED

No point setting a goal unless there's no action plan to go with it. Make a list of things you're going to do to attain your goal, both - long and short-term.

Consider the action you're going to take to overcome any anticipated obstacles.

A sample list of action-oriented weight loss goals might look like this:

Drink a full glass of water every two hours (set alarm).

Walk home instead of driving three times a week - Monday, Wednesday, and Friday.

Remove refined sugar from the house; replaced with Raw Honey & Coconut Nectar

Some of the obstacles you may face, would be things like setbacks and trigger situations. Plan to take care of them in advance; when you **"Anticipate"** such things, they are a lot of less likely to ruin your efforts and strip you of motivation.

Review your action plan periodically, and note what works and what doesn't, and why. Adjust as needed.

Step 4: REALISTIC

Unreasonable expectations - the main reason people fail (at weight loss, and many other things in life). Unreasonable expectations result in disappointment, which usually leads to de-motivation.

By living a Sedentary lifestyle, lack of willpower, food addiction laziness etc... All these things are nothing compared to the destructive nature of de-motivation. It must be avoided at all costs.

That is why it's so important to set SMART weight loss goals. Unrealistic goals are guaranteed to result in de-motivation, which means not only that you will fail with your current weight loss plan, but also that it will be more difficult to embark on one in the future due to emotional barriers.

Basically: if you want to stay motivated (which is essential for successful weight loss), your goals must be realistic. **How do you make sure that your goals are realistic? Consider this:**

You did not end up at your current weight overnight, so you will not lose it overnight.

How far are you prepared to go? How bad do you want to slim down and how fast do you want it? Are you ready to work extra hard -- for extra results, or are you not in a hurry?

What can you expect from your chosen method? Are you going to use extreme methods for rapid weight loss, or employ a more 'slow and steady' approach?

What is your body capable of? If you're pear-shaped, you must understand that losing weight will not change the genetically predetermined structure of your body. You must understand that the stubborn fat in problem areas is going to be the last to disappear.

If a goal is physically attainable, it does not mean it's realistic. A goal is 'realistic' when you believe that it can be attained — Know your limits

Step 5: TIMED

You must set a timeframe for each goal. Creating a time frame also creates a sense of urgency, so your mind is more likely to urge your body to complete the goal when it's due in a specific amount of time.

Work towards a "realistic" deadlines.

Don't says: "I want to lose weight sometime soon."

Do says: "I will drop a dress size by the end of next week."

Incorporate this goal setting strategy into your weight loss plan, and see how it affects its efficiency.

Chapter 2

Why Are You Gaining Weight?

Health Issues behind Weight Gain

Weight gains are often associated with food intake. Why are we suffer a sudden increase in weight despite the tremendous effort put on dieting and exercising, some of the health conditions and diseases can be the reasons for the weight gain?

There are Five Common Health Conditions for your thorough understanding, should consult and take necessary action to seek professional advice & treatment.

1. Cushing's syndrome

Cortisol is an essential hormone of our body that is being produced by the adrenal glands. Cushing's syndrome developed due to an overproduction of cortisol.

Cortisol imbalanced can cause weight gain very quickly — our Body Fluid retention in the tissues and trigger, which causes the weight gain of a person.

People who are suffering from this kind of condition have the characteristic of a "**Round Shaped Face**".

Signs and symptoms are;

Frequent urination
Feeling of thirst
Reduced libido or lack of sexual appetite
Some psychological problems in women, the menstrual period becomes
 irregular
Buffalo hump on the neck or shoulders
Arms and legs are often not proportion
Spots on the face chest or shoulder

Headaches
Back pain
Skin darkening on the neck
Skin becomes thinner and easily bruised
Bruises and scratches, as well as insect bites, take time to heal
Reddish-purple stretch marks found in the abdomen, buttocks, arms, legs
 or breast

2. Essential Fatty Acid Deficiency

Our body requires essential fatty acids for metabolic functions, deficiency

in fatty acids in the body would trigger one to crave for High in Fat Foods.

Common Signs and symptoms are;

Poor wound healing
Dandruff
Dry hair
Dry and scaly skin
Mouth ulcers
Increased susceptibility to infection

Essential Fatty Acid Deficiency may cause the following health conditions:

Arthritis
Eczema
Heart disease
diabetes
Premenstrual syndrome

3. Food Sensitivity

Food allergic and can cause itchiness on skin appearance. Food sensitivity effect of the allergen taken into the body may not be immediate. A symptom like a body swelling, weight gain may be observed right after the allergic attack.

Signs and symptoms experience from food sensitivity:

Heartburn
Headache
Indigestion fatigue
Depression
Joint pain
Canker sore
Chronic respiratory symptom

4. Hypothyroidism

Our body may insufficiently produce the hormone thyroid by the thyroid gland. Thyroid hormone regulates the metabolism. When the Thyroid hormones are low, the body slows down of the body's metabolism.

It could either cause a loss in appetite or gain weight.

The cause of weight gain is due to the fluid retention caused by protein deposits in the body.

Signs and symptoms are;

Dry skin
Coarse skin
Decreased sweating
Poor memory
Slow speech
Hoarse voice
Weakness
Headache
Intolerance to cold
Fatigue
Lethargy or sleepiness
Swelling on the face or around the eyes

5. Prescription Drugs

Research has shown that people who use Prescription Medication daily can cause an increase in the appetite of a person.

Oral contraceptives in women could also cause fluid to be retained in the body, thus bloating and increase in weight. Due to the change in hormones, some women may suffer from mood swing, depression for some women.

Chapter 3

Weight Loss and Nutrition

Proper Nutrition For Desired Weight Loss

An effective weight loss program begins with proper nutrition. Most people believe that restricting nutritious calories will somehow lead to their desired weight loss. But this is not only dangerous to your body but have proven to be untrue.

So what is so important about nutrition, and how does it relate to weight loss?

Well, the answer to this question can be answered in very simple terms. If you feed your body the proper nutrition, you will feel for the longer, and will be less likely to overeat. Proper nutrition also fuels your metabolism. If you eat the right foods at the right times your metabolism will increase and your body will become more efficient at burning fat.

Let's look at the five basic components of food recently. The five essential elements of food are carbohydrates, proteins, fats, vitamins, and minerals. All are needed in order to provide your body with proper Carbohydrates

Foods containing carbohydrates are potatoes, fruits, vegetables, and whole grains. Starchy foods and sugar are converted by the body into glucose, and this is the body's main fuel source. Foods that are derived from plants are the best source of carbohydrates because the body takes some time to break down the starch into glucose and this prevents your body's sugar level from spiking or dropping to dramatically.

Eating highly refined foods usually converts to glucose to quickly in the bloodstream and this can lead to an overactive or worn out pancreas, which can lead to diabetes. An additional benefit of deriving your carbohydrates from plant-based foods is the fact that these foods are usually high in fiber. Fiber is a bulking agent which helps to keep the undigested food in the interest constantly on the move. And this will prevent constipation and other gastric issues.

Fad diets lack the proper nutritional value and thus do not offer any long time solutions for weight loss. Healthy nutrition is a must when you are looking forward to some effective solutions.

Try to incorporate fruits and vegetables into your diet as much as possible. You can take a mixture of fresh veggies in salad while having dinner; berries can be added to the breakfast cereal. Vegetables can replace unhealthy French fries from your meals. The canned vegetables can be replaced with frozen varieties. Foods of different colours offer different kinds of nutrients to the diet. Make sure you are incorporating fruits and veggies of all colours like green, white, yellow, orange and red.

Whole grains constitute healthy nutritional diet. The foods rich in whole grain include rice, noodles, bread. In the western cultures, use of quinoa, barley is very common. When you shop for whole wheat bread, you need to be well aware of the contents in the food. See the nutritional contents well and check that cereals or bread are not made of plain wheat flour. On the other hand, whole wheat flour is richer in nutritional status.

Apart from the incorporation of these healthy food options mentioned above, it is extremely essential to limit the intake of fatty foods and sugary substances for effective weight loss. Intake of fat from good sources like canola oil and olive oil is beneficial for your health. Stay away from saturated fats, butter if you want to cut down on the levels of trans fat. Increase intake of whole, fresh foods.

You can gain weight even when you are overeating the good foods, so make sure you are eating healthy. You must keep a check on the total calorie count and for this you can get in touch with a nutritionist who can prepare a customized diet chart for you.

High Protein Foods

What High Protein Foods Are Healthy and Help to Lose Weight?

Foods rich in protein help you lose weight. How? Very simple. Protein builds muscle and muscle in turn burns fat. You probably have heard that many times from personal trainers and if you haven't, now you know. If you want to lose weight, it is very important to eat diet high in protein along with fruits and vegetables. Don't forget about complex carbohydrates either. Do not eat simple carbs like pizza, white pasta and white sugar. Instead nourish your body with complex carbohydrates like brown rice, sprouted bread and fruits.

So what are high protein foods that help you lose weight? There are two major sources of protein: animal and vegetable based. The name says it all. The first one, animal based protein, is sourced from animals. For example: Chicken breast, Lean Beef, Cheese & Butter, Seafood, etc. Vegetable sources of protein consist of of quinoa, beans, tofu, seaweed / kelp, Green salad etc.

Sweet foods rich in carb which is good for sugar craving

One of the things that people struggle with when trying to lose weight are cravings for unhealthy foods. Well, I have good news, there are certain foods that will help you fight off those cravings and help you burn fat at the same. Even better, these are foods you are going to like. They are very sweet, so they can fix your craving for sugar while providing you other beneficial nutrients too.

Fruit: Berries and Tomatoes and more *see below tables

Vegetable: like Carrot, Red Capsaican

Legumes: like lentils, beans and chickpeas

Dark Chocolate

Sweet Potatoes

Nuts

Sugar-Free Chewing Gum or Mints

FRUITS Products:	Size	Calories	Protein (g)
Banana	½ cup	69	0.8
Watermelon	½ cup	24.3	0.5
Apricot	½ cup	39.6	1.2
Strawberry	½ cup	25	0.5
Cantalope	½ cup	27.3	0.7
Apple	½ cup	36.9	0.1
Orange	½ cup	42.3	0.8

Type of Carbohydrate foods to avoid

Carbohydrate is the prime source of energy. But not all carbs are created equal, especially when it comes to rapid weight loss. And the difference between good and bad carbs can transform your body.

These are the list of Carbohydrate foods you should avoid if you want to lose weight:

Refined Cereals

Beer

Barbecue Sauce

White Pasta

White Bread

White Rice

Deep Fried food &Chips

Processed & Cured Meat

Candy Snacks and Gummies

Cake and dessert

The weight loss program is all about enjoying the fun of eating nutritional foods. With an improved diet plan, you can find your energies reaching new heights. You feel light as well as positive. Even if you find the lifestyle changes hard to maintain in the initial phases, it is essential to focus on your goals and enjoy your new dietary habits in order to get the desired results out of your hardwork.

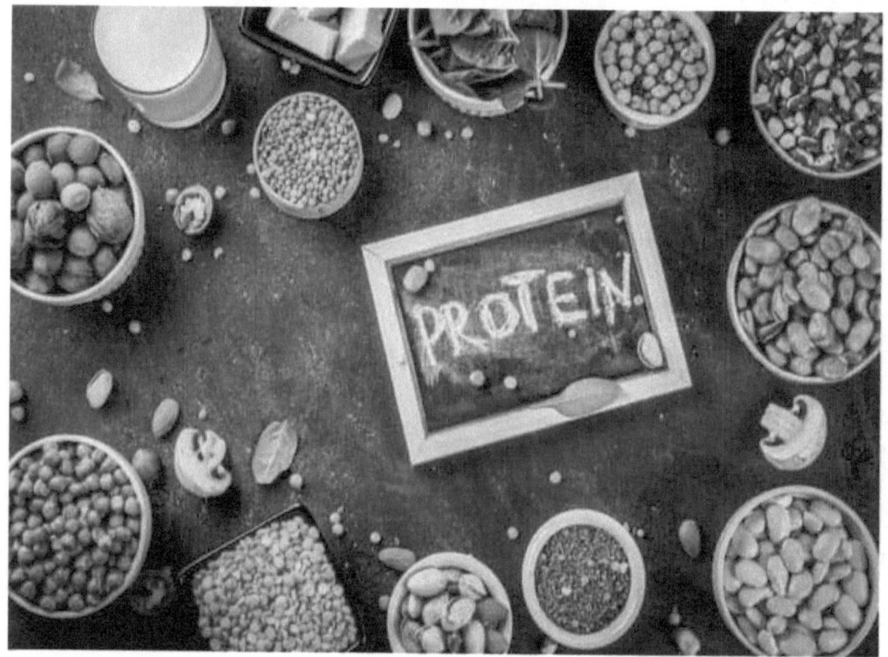

Chapter 4

How t0 Cleanse the Body for Weight Loss

A Successful Weight Loss Diet Starts from the Inside!

If you're like most people, you've been on a million weight loss diets, from Weight Watchers and Atkins to South Beach and celeb diets. You voraciously read magazines for their weight loss tips and gravitate toward the headlines that promise you can lose weight fast. The chances are good that you to have, indeed, lost weight on many of these diets, but the chances are even better that you've gained it all back - plus some.

Weight Loss Diet Failure

You've probably bought into the propaganda that says you've failed at dieting; a different — and more accurate - way of looking at it is that the weight loss diet has failed you. That's because most diets focus on short-term changes that result in temporary weight loss, but never tackle the underlying factors that make you put on the pounds to begin with.

In other words, they focus only on the "outside" problem - your body - and neglect everything below the surface - your emotions, your intellect, and your relationships. A diet for summer might work but you can bet by winter it will be back to haunt you again.

Turning Failure into Success

In order to lose weight and keep it off, you need a guide who will lead you on an exploratory journey to discover the power and control that you possess. Then, you need to be taught how to harness those powers to achieve all that you want in life - including fitting into your jeans again.

You may have been told - either verbally or through insidious advertisements - that if you don't have power over your eating, you have no power at all. Nothing could be further from the truth. Every Person is magnificent, and every person has mental powers, emotional powers, social powers and physical powers just waiting to be tapped. When you heal your past wounds, and recognize and reinforce the power within you, you have laid the foundation for permanent weight loss.

So in the following chapters, I will show you how to lose weight effortlessly.

Over come Your Plateau with Easy Tips

If you need to lose a few extra pounds but feel you've hit a plateau, there are several ways to get your body back in the weight loss mode. A plateau is when you're no longer losing weight though it seems nothing has changed in your diet or exercise routine. Your body has adapted to the diet and now refuses to budge. So you must make some changes to boost your weight loss again.

These 4 weight loss tips can help;

1. Change your calorie intake.

One way to overcome a plateau while maintaining a healthy weight loss plan is to change your calorie intake. Monitor how many calories you're eating and decrease them slightly to see if your weight scale moves again. You might try the zigzag method as well. To do this, decrease calories one day, and then increase calories the next. This helps shift your body out of its comfort zone. Only make minor adjustments and monitor your weight with each small change.

2. Replace a snack or two.

If you usually eat a chocolate bar as a mid-afternoon snack, try replacing this with a fruit or vegetable. Eat apples, bananas, carrots and low-fat dip, or celery and low-fat dip instead of chocolate. Fruits and vegetables are not only filling, but they also promote healthy weight loss.

3. Keep exercising, but endure longer.

Another way to boost weight loss and get your body moving again is to increase your exercise time. Instead of 30 minutes a day, try exercising 45 minutes a day. Walk every chance you get. Walking is a great (non-strenuous) exercise that helps your heart and promotes healthy weight loss. Park your car a little farther from the mall than usual when shopping. Walk your dog twice a day instead of only once. Take a walk during your breaks at work. These small changes can make a big difference in your weight loss efforts.

4. Monitor "what" you are eating.

Are you eating mainly sugar and carbohydrates on your weight loss diet? If so, try replacing one or two of these with a protein-rich food. Protein is a proven fat burner and energy booster, and many weight trainers use it to boost their workouts. Protein also helps you fill full longer so you're less likely to be hungry an hour later. There are protein snack bars on the market now so you can easily get a boost during the day. Other changes you can make include increasing your water and fibre intake if you feel you're not getting enough of these.

How to Choose a Weight Loss Plan

Whether you need to lose only a few extra Kg's or up to 20 or 60kg's, you can become weary while trying to choose among the hundreds of weight loss plans available. There are plenty of weight loss diets that involve eating special foods, drinking certain drink mixtures, or taking weight loss pills. But which one's right for you? Use these tips to choose the weight loss diet that will fit your lifestyle and daily routine.

What is Your Style?

A weight loss diet plan should fit your style. What works for one person may or may not work for you. You must consider your daily routine, the types of foods you like, and what your body needs. Do you enjoy sweets? Do you enjoy eating meats?

There are a number of diets that allow you to eat meats and sweets in moderation. Also, consider how many meals you can eat. Do you normally eat three square meals per day, or do you take smaller, more frequent meals? These are questions to ask before starting a weight loss plan so you can find a diet that's easy to stay with to reach your goals.

Study the Risks

Some diets are more risky than others when it comes to weight loss and your health. For instance, fast weight loss can be harmful to the body, especially if continued over a long period of time. Weight loss pills can be dangerous too if taken without first consulting a physician. Some diets are harmful to the body if you have certain health conditions.

For instance, a diet that emphasizes meat might not be best if you already have digestive problems or heart problems. If you have any serious health problems or are taking prescription medications, you should talk with your doctor before starting a weight loss diet.

Types of Weight Loss Diets

There are many weight loss plans, but each is different. It's a good idea to study the different types of plans before getting started on your weight loss journey. Find the variety of weight loss diet that best suits you. Consider how each affects your body and health, and how each plan fits into your schedule or routine. Let's see what types of diet plans are available and what is required with each.

Diets for Fast Weight Loss

Though fast weight loss is not recommended for the long term, there are some quick diets to help you lose 2-6kgs in no time. These include the low-carb diet, three-to-five-day meal replacement shakes, water or juice fasts, and alternate vegetable/fruit diets in which you eat only fruits one day and only vegetables the next. These diets work great for a quick fix but are very difficult (and possibly unhealthy) to maintain for the long term.

Low Calorie Weight Loss Diets

There are many low calorie diets with which you will reduce your daily calories to lose weight. There are several ways to monitor your calories. You can read food labels and count the calories of everything you eat. You can also use a calorie guide to determine how many calories are in certain foods or dishes that do not have labels. Weight Watchers provides an easy point counter that calculates points based on calories, fiber, and fat grams in foods.

Fixed Menu Plans

With a fixed menu diet plan, you will be given a list of all the foods you can eat. The meal plans are put together especially for you based on your likes and needs. This type of diet can make things easy for you as you lose weight, but keep in mind that you will eventually need to start planning your own meals again. So it's a good idea to learn how to plan your meals after you've lost the initial weight. This will help you keep the weight off once the fixed-menu diet has ended.

Exchange Food Diet

With an exchange food diet, you will plan meals with a set number of servings from several food groups. The foods are determined by calorie intake, and you can pick and choose among foods that have the same calories to give you a variety of choices at each meal. This diet is great if you've just completed a fixed menu diet because it allows you to make your own food choices each day.

Low Fat Diet

Another type of diet is the low fat diet, which requires lowering the intake of fat. This doesn't mean eating fat-free everything but merely reducing fats (especially saturated fats) and oils to a normal level according to the food pyramid. Fat should take up around 30 percent of the calories eaten. Lowering saturated fat promotes healthy weight loss and helps lower cholesterol levels to promote good heart health. There are many foods that advertise "low fat" but many of these are also very high in sugar. Look for foods that are low in fat and low in sugar for healthy weight loss. Also, limit fast foods or make healthier choices from the menu such as salads or grilled foods. Many fried fast foods are loaded with fat.

Weight Loss through Reduced Portions

There are also weight loss diets with which only the portions are reduced, but you basically eat anything you want. You eats only small portions of foods and basically follow your stomach. When your stomach is empty, you eat slowly until you feel satisfied, but not overly full. You only eat when you're really hungry. This type of diet gives you freedom to choose what you want to eat, but limits how much you can eat. The concept is when you eat less food in smaller portions then you're also eating less fat and calories with every meal, no matter what the food.

There are also pre-packaged meals and formulas to help promote weight loss. Almost any diet can work if you adhere to its rules, add activity or exercises, and drink plenty of water. Study each type of diet to find one that will work for you, and check with you doctor before starting a new diet plan if you have a health condition or take medications. You can easily research diet plans online and find many free weight loss tips to help you develop a plan.

Natural Detox Strategies to Cleanse

Your Body

We are all exposed to a high number of environmental pollutants, including man-made chemicals on a daily basis. Harmful substances that infiltrate the body can also come from consumption of processed and fast food, high sugar diets, medications, poor quality drinking water, personal care items, household products, and more.

It is no wonder our body has a hard time keeping things balanced. When we are full of toxins and impurities, it is difficult to lose weight. From time to time, we require a good "house cleaning" on the inside. Detoxification promotes a wide range of health advantages.

During and after the process, you'll enjoy these benefits

1. **Cleanse the Body:** The number one benefit of detoxing is allowing the body to rid itself of any excess waste it's been storing. Allowing toxins need to exit the body can benefit every organ and function.

2. **Boost in Energy:** Individuals engaging in a detox frequently report feeling more energetic. This would make sense because while you're detoxing you are cleansing your body of damaging substances to increase proper functioning of all your systems.

3. **Unhealthy Food Addiction:** If you have addictions to sugar, caffeine, fried, or other unhealthy foods that are filled with empty calories, you can use a detox program to help you kill those cravings. Often if you just try to quit eating those foods or drinking those beverages "cold turkey," you'll have limited success and go back to your old ways. But if you cleanse the body and replace those foods with healthier choices, you can retrain yourself.

4. **Weight Loss Support:** Beginning a weight loss program with detoxification can immediately provide improvement in eating habits and a feeling of lightness. When you stops eating foods that weigh you down, a lighter feeling is bound to occur.

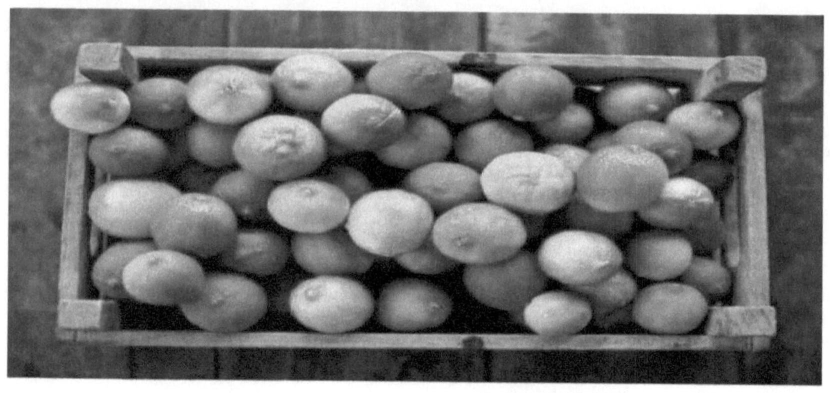

How to detox your body naturally
In Six Easy Step

Step One: Five Super Food

Choosing a balanced and essential foods to a successful detox.

GINGER, LIME, RAW HONEY, MATCHA, CAYENNE PEPPER & TURMERIC POWER all contain beneficial antioxidants which are molecules that help protects cell health, slow down aging and guard against health concerns. Amazingly food sources to beat your weight gain issue.

Ginger, Lime with Raw Honey Tea

The Citric acids from Lime are suitable for boosting body metabolism, reduces body fat and excessive calories; hence, it is practical for weight control.

Lime contains high in Flavonoids are phytochemicals that are for favorable for treating metabolic disorders. Properties to improve body inflammatory, diabetic, and cancer-fighting.

Both Lime & Ginger Roots is high in Vitamin C and magnesium. Ginger tea with honey and Lime juice make a great soothing beverage. Improve digestion and battling stomach bloating symptom.

Both Lime & Ginger is also high in antioxidants properties to improve body immunity and has a calming effect on healing and relieve stress.

Ginger had long been recognised and heavily used in cooking, baking, soup and beverages in many parts of the world.

Ginger is high in amino acids, which help to improve blood circulation and boost body metabolism to help promote Burning of Calories in our body. This Superfood comes with many benefits include: Relieve nausea,

Ginger contains anti-inflammatory properties to help aids joints and muscle ache and pain.

Preparation time 3 minutes

1 tablespoons of lime juice

1 tablespoons of ginger juice

half tablespoons of Raw Honey

Mixed all ingredient into One glass of warm water

 # Tips: to pre-prepared Lime & Ginger in one setting

Preparation time: 30 minutes

300 grams of Lime

300 grams of Ginger root

Half cup of warm water

Washed both ingredients cut into small wedges, put all the ingredient in the Blender with skin on. Blend till all the ingredients are broken down to juice.

Squeeze, filter the juice and make ice cube. 2 tablespoon per ice cube

---

Nature Detox Supplements

Matcha Power (Green Tea) – Boost Metabolism

Cayenne Chili Pepper Power – Suppress Hunger

Turmeric Power – Liver cleansing

Guideline for the in-take of supplements according to weight size.

Weight size	Capsules per day	Matcha	Tumeric	Cayenne Pepper
50 -80 kgs	Breakfast	3	2	2
	Lunch	3	2	2
	Dinner		2	2
90 - 120kgs	Breakfast	4	3	3
	Lunch	4	3	3
	Dinner		3	3
130 - 160kgs	Breakfast	5	4	4
	Lunch	5	4	4
	Dinner		4	4

*If your body over-reactive to high doses, try to reduce the number of capsules and continue to monitor your system. If discomfort persists stop immediately.

The combination of the Detox Tea and Detox Supplements will enhance weight loss and weight maintenance in people who are overweight and moderately obese.

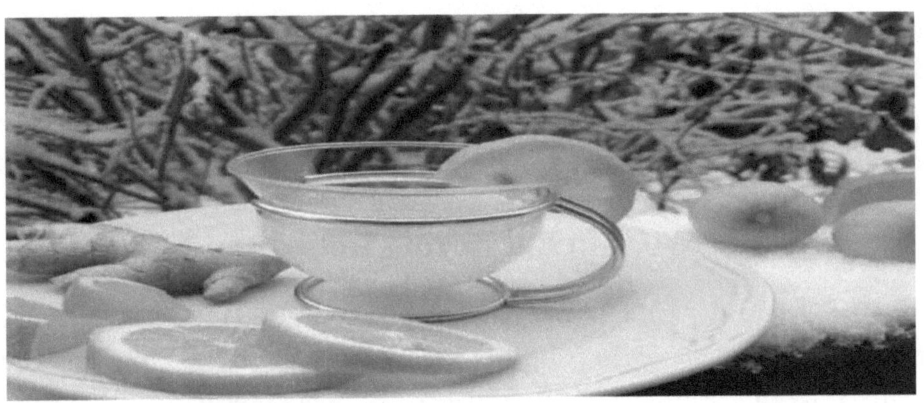

Step 2: Follow Superfood Detox Routine

Upon waking: Drink a Glass of warm Ginger Lime with raw honey tea first thing in the morning before consuming any food.

Before Breakfast pop – Matcha, Cayenne Pepper & Turmeric

Lunch: Drink a Glass of warm Ginger Lime with raw honey tea before consuming any food together with **– Matcha, Cayenne Pepper & Turmeric**

Evening: Drink a Glass of warm Ginger Lime with raw honey tea before consuming any food

A good way to end the day is to eliminate toxins with **Cayenne Pepper & Turmeric** *two hours prior to bedtime to assure a good night's rest.*

Hint:

Rinse your mouth after the Ginger Lime with raw honey tea to prevent our teeth enamel corrode by the acid.

Duration of this Superfood Detox Routine: 14 Days

Detox our body regularly can re-condition our body system by remove toxicity, cleanse gut and better nutrients absorption.

Suggest at least 14 Days or even up to 28 Days, along with a GREEN FOOD DIET.

Hint: Detoxing should be done at least 3-4 times per year for an Overall Health & Weight Maintenance.

Step 3: What to Eat during Detox Routine

One of the greatest benefits of detoxification compared to a fasting cleanse is that you can (and should) eat healthy foods throughout the program. The objective is to increasing pH level and re-condition body system.

Since the goal is to detoxify your body, you want to consume the healthiest, most organic foods possible, after all is only for 14 days ☺

Below are some Guidelines & Menu Plan to guide you during this Detox process:

1. Fruits and Vegetables

Leafy greens (such as kale and spinach) and cruciferous vegetables (such as broccoli, cauliflower and brussel sprouts), are especially detox-friendly since they are low in calories and carbohydrates, but loaded with fiber. Sticking with fruits and vegetables even after the detox program is a good way to keep toxins moving out of the body. Eat them raw whenever possible.

Certified organic produce assures it has been grown without pesticides, synthetic fertilizers, sewage sludge, genetically modified organisms or ionizing radiation. Organic fruits and vegetables have the healthiest nutritional profile possible and the least amount of toxins. After all, the goal of a detoxification program is to rid the body of harmful chemicals.

2. Fats

Most people are shocked to learn that fats should be part of their daily diet. However, all fats are not created equal. Focus on only fats from healthy sources such as fish high in Omega oil, olive oil, avocados, nuts and coconut oil.

3. Proteins

Lean proteins that are low in saturated fat should be the only type consumed during a tea detox. Again, consider organic sources of eggs, poultry, fish and other food. Vegetarian proteins such as spinach, beans and quinoa are also healthy protein options.

4. Fibre

This often overlooked item is crucial to a successful weight loss program. It is the ingredient that creates a feeling of "fullness" and aids in the movement of food, assisting the body in eliminating toxins. Good sources of fibre are vegetables, fruits, beans and nuts.

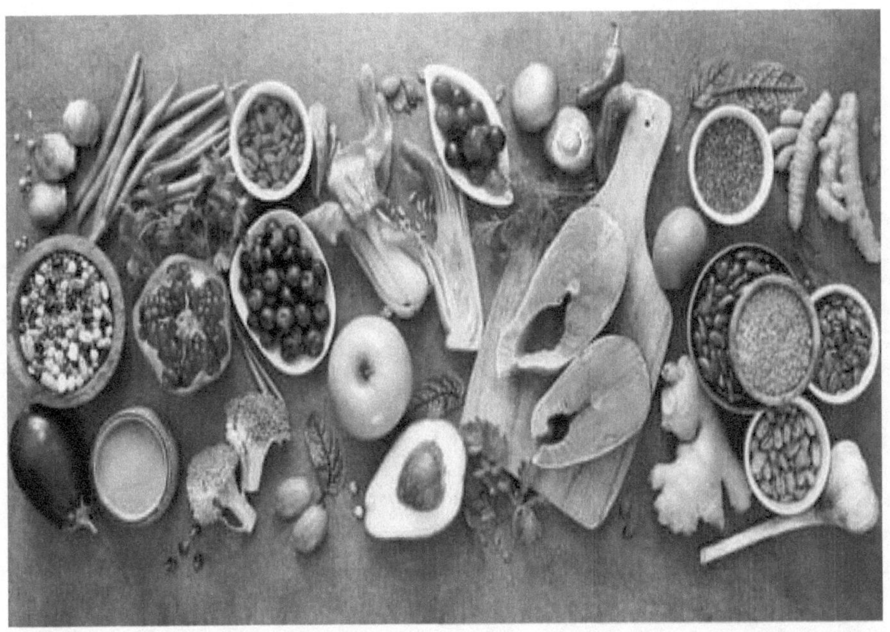

Step 4: Green Food Recipes

TEN GREEN FOOD RECIPES FOR YOU TO COMBINE WITH YOUR DETOX ROUTINE

Below menu is focus on Lean Protein to help replenish Alkaline in your body system to support and improve Weight loss effectively.

The menu portions are varied, advice you to eat according to your normal daily consumption portion, it will be better to follow the

"Rule of Thumbs "method to plan your meal accordingly.

Rule of the Thumbs

Breakfast – Eat like a KING

Lunch – Eat Moderately

Dinner – Eat like a POOR Man *Last meal hour before 8pm*

Remember to Drink 6 – 8 glass of water each day

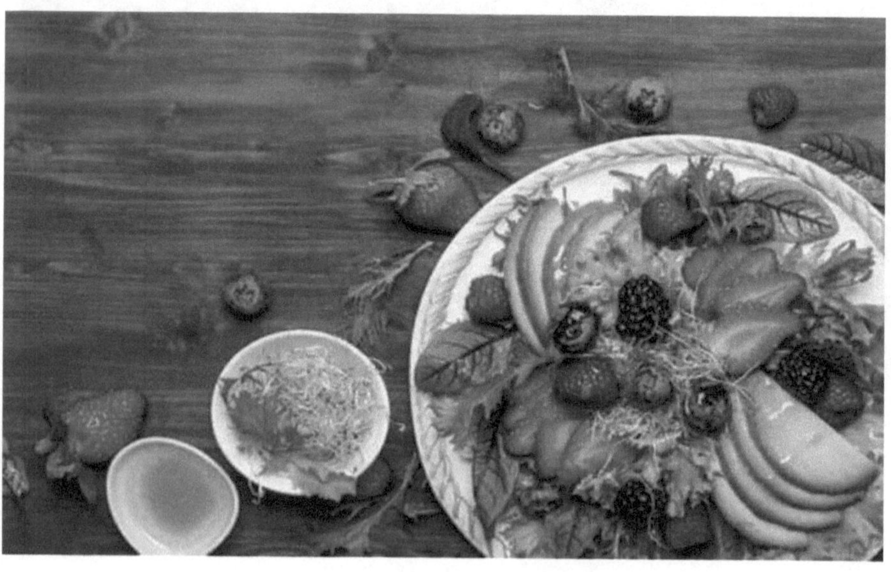

Baked Pumpkin with sweet potaotes

Serving : 4

Preparation time : 15 minutes

Cooking time : 15 minutes

Calories 600 Protein 9

3 cups of Steam Mashed Pumpkin   (Calories 147, Protein 5.4)

Half cups of Steam Mashed Sweet Potatoes   (Calories 103, Protein 1.7)

Half cup of Crated Carrot   (Calories 35 , Protein 0.9)

Half cup of Mashed Banana   (Calories 69 , Protein 0.8)

2 Tablespoon of Virgin Coconut Oil   (Calories 240, Protein 0)

Half teaspoon of Cinnamon power & a pinch Pink Salt

One Tablespoon of Corn starch

Turn on the Oven 200 deg C, set the time 15 minutes

Oil the 8 inches size Baking Tin with some coconut oil

Assemble all the Ingredients mixed well, place it in the oven.

#Tips

This is a perfect meal on its own;

*Can spread one palm size of Toasted Pumpkin seed on the slice of Baked Sweet
Potatoes with coconut yogurt. Is also a great energy treats for anytime of the day.*

Chia seed Parfait

***Soak Half cup of Chia seed with water leave in the fridge overnight**

Serving : 1

Preparation time : 10 minutes

Calories 363 Protein 18.5

Chia seed – 1 oz, 85g   (Calories 138, Protein 5)

Strawberries) ½ cup   (Calories 25, Protein 0.5)

Coconut Nectar syrup – 1 tablespoon   (Calories 50, Protein 0)

Plain Coconut Yogurt - 150 g   (Calories 150, Protein 13)

(Mixed few dash of Cinnamon power)

Assemble – Mixed Yogurt with coconut nectar and lay each ingredient in a few layers.
**Chia seed soaked with water and leave in the fridge overnight

Drizzle Coconut Nectar over the top and savor!

Avocado with Brown rice cracker "Taco"

Serving : 1

Preparation time : 10 minutes

Total : Calories 190g Protein 9.5g

Brown Rice cracker 2 pieces   (Calories 38 , Protein 4.4)

Half Medium size Avocado   (Calories 125, Protein 4)

Half cup Cherry Tomatoes   (Calories 19, Protein 0.8)

Avocado chop, Seasons with some Pink salt, pepper, Lime juice

Balsamic reduction vinegar on top of avocado.

Great Energy Booster meal will set your morning right!

Waldorf Salad

Serving : 1

Preparation time : 15 minutes

Cooking time : 15 minutes

Total : Calories 276g Protein 7.31

Half cup of Boil Potatoes into cube size   (Calories 83, Protein 2.91)

One cup Apple –chopped to bite size   (Calories 74, Protein 0.2)

Half cup Celery - chopped to bite size   (Calories 14.3, Protein 0.)

35g Crushed Toasted Almond nuts   (Calories 67, Protein 2)

1/4 cup (37.5g) Plain Coconut Yogurt   (Calories 37.5, Protein 2.2)

One Teaspoon - Lime Juice

Add: Pepper, Himalayan Pink Salt. Olive oil to taste.

Assemble all the ingredients and place in the fridge.

This Salad great for Lunch and Dinner, taste delicious in chilled temperature.

Soba Combo

Serving : 1

Preparation time : 15 minutes

Cooking time : 10 minutes

Total : Calories 215g Protein 63.5g

1. *Buckwheat noodle 1 cup 114g*   *(Calories 113. Protein 58)*

    Boil of Pot of water, drop the noodle into the water once it's boiled

    Cooked the noodle till al-dente (5 to 8 mins - checking by breaking one string)

    Prepare a bowl of cold water to rinse the noodle, drained and set aside.

2. *Half cup Japanese cucumber*   *(Calories 6.8. Protein 0.4)*

    Washed and cut the cucumber into bite size, place in a small bowl

3. *Light soya vinegar dressing*   *(Calories 70. Protein 4)*

    2 tablespoon of premium quality light soya sauce (Calories 16. Protein 2)

    One teaspoon of Japanese rice vinegar (Calories 15. Protein 0)

    Half teaspoon of Bloody Orange Marmalade

    Half teaspoon Sesame oil

4. *Instant Miso soup with seaweed / Nori*   *(Calories 25. Protein 1)*

    Soup bowl mixed the Miso soup with boil water

Toss the noodle, cucumber and dressing in a mixing bowl, plate it a top with roasted nori.

This a perfect meal for Lunch or Dinner

Sweet & sour Tofu mixed Veggie Salad

Serving : 1

Preparation time : 30 minutes

Cooking time: 5 minutes

Total : Calories 458.3g Protein 21.4g

1. Extra Firm Tofu 85g   *(Calories 150. Protein 16)*

   Cut into cube, pan fried with vegetable oil till golden

2. Half cup Fresh chopped Turnip   *(Calories 18. Protein 1.5)*

3. Half cup chopped Japanese Cucumber   *(Calories 6.8. Protein 0.4)*

4. Toasted Chopped Cashew nuts 42g   *(Calories 80. Protein 2)*

5. Dressing   *(Calories 100. Protein 0.5)*

   Blood orange marmalade – 2 tablespoons *(Calories 70. Protein 0.5)*

   Cayenne chili powder – 1 teaspoon   *(Calories 13. Protein 0.5)*

   lime juice – 2 teaspoons   *(Calories 3. Protein 0)*

   sesame oil – 1/2 teaspoon   *(Calories 17.5. Protein 0)*

Pink salt to taste

This is a fantastic light dinner to end your day!

Sir Fried Mixed Cruciferous

Serving : 1

Preparation time : 15 minutes

Cooking time : 15 minutes

Total : Calories 210 g Protein 14.4g

1. One Cup – Broccoli, Cut to desire size   *(Calories 43.6. Protein 4.6)*

2. One Cup – Cauliflower, Cut to desire size   *(Calories 28.6. Protein 2.2)*

3. *Half cup – cooked de-shelled Edamame*   *(Calories 95. Protein 6)*

4. One cup Red Bell Pepper, dice to small pieces *(Calories 28. Protein 1.6)*

   4 thin slices of ginger

   1 teaspoon - Mushroom food enhancer power

   1 tablespoon of Vegetable oil

   Pink salt and pepper to taste.

Steam Broccoli & Cauliflower for 5 minutes

Heat the Frying Pan, add in Oil & Ginger, stir in the Bell Pepper, fry till is soft and put in both veggies combine all the ingredients and add in the seasoning with 2 tablespoons of water to let it simmer for 3 minutes.

This is a perfect stress-free healthy meal to eat on its own.

Boiled Broccoli & Sauté mushroom w garlic & herbs

Serving : 1

Preparation time : 15 minutes

Cooking time : 15 minutes

Total : Calories 260g Protein 11g

(A) One & ½ Cup – Broccoli, Cut to desire size   *(Calories 65.4. Protein 6.9)*

4 thin slices of ginger

1 teaspoon of Vegetable oil

Half Teaspoon – Pink salt

Boil a Pot of water add in all ingredient let Broccoli simmer for 5 – 8 minutes.

(B) 1 cup of Button Mushroom quarter in size   *(Calories 42.2. Protein 3.4)*

2 cloves of finely chopped Garlic

1 tablespoon of chopped white onion

1 tablespoon of finely chopped Coriander

1 tablespoon of Olive oil   *(Calories 133, Protein 0)*

Pink salt and pepper to taste.

Heat the Frying Pan, add in Oil & Garlic, fry till fragrant and golden, remove all ingredient from the Pan.

Put the Mushroom into the same Pan fry with NO Oil, till is fragrant and soft.

Last assemble all ingredient – Garlic oil, herbs and seasoning.

This is a Hearty meal can goes will with Miso soup or just on its own.

Step 5: Food to Avoid

There are certain foods and substances that must be avoided during a weight loss detox, such as sugar and alcohol. Become aware of how destructive these type of man-made substances can be to your overall health. They can destroy your weight loss efforts. The following are the foods you should try to avoid during the tea detoxification process:

Sugary foods and beverages: If you have a sweet tooth, you should try to curb it. Not only is sugar bad for your teeth, but it also fills your body with toxins. The only sugar you should be eating is from natural food.

Processed food: Much of the toxic load in our bodies comes from eating processed food including highly-processed fast food. If there are ingredients on the label you cannot pronounce, stay away from it.

Most Grains: Even whole grains cause a rapid rise in blood sugar which triggers insulin secretion. Bread, baked goods and pastas can encourage weight gain. They should be limited during your detox.

Artificial Sweeteners: These has no place in a healthy diet. Avoid aspartame, saccharin, sucralose, cyclamates and others. Use all-natural sweeteners instead.

Alcohol: No matter how much you enjoy it, you must acknowledge that alcohol is not part of a healthy lifestyle.

Step 6: Improve your success

There are a few other actions you can undertake to achieve your goal of weight loss.

1. Sleep

Numerous studies demonstrate that lack of sleep can seriously affect your weight negatively. In fact, many experts believe sleep controls your diet.

Sleeping less than five hours a night actually promotes weight gain.

Sleep deprivation increases preferences for high-calorie foods and overall calorie intake.

Individuals who slept less than six hours a were more likely to gain 11 pounds compared with participants who slept seven hours a night.

Not sleeping enough can reduce and undo the benefits of dieting, cancelling out all the hard work of weight loss.

Sleep duration appears to affect the hormones regulating hunger and can stimulate a person's appetite. When you're short on sleep, you are more tempted to skip exercise, make poor food choices and become irritable.

2. Body Massage & Foot Reflexology

Study has proven that both Body Massage and Foot Reflexology will promote better blood circulation to burn fat and water retention issue. Improve in overall health wellbeing. Both have therapeutic effect and can effectively releases body stress and help to enhance sleeping quality.

3. Exercise

We now live in a sedentary culture and studies show all that sitting is taking a significant toll on our health. Prolonged sitting at your desk or in the car, playing video games or watching television negatively impacts cardiovascular and metabolic function and is increasing our waistlines.

Dr. James Levine from the Mayo Clinic has empathically stated that, "Sitting is more dangerous than smoking, kills more people than HIV and is more treacherous than parachuting. We are sitting ourselves to death. Science has also discovered that many toxic elements appeared to be excreted through sweat, lending support to the benefits of exercise in a detoxification program.

With any weight loss program, you have to move. It does not have to be a trip to the gym. Dancing, walking to the store, gardening, mall walking…it counts.

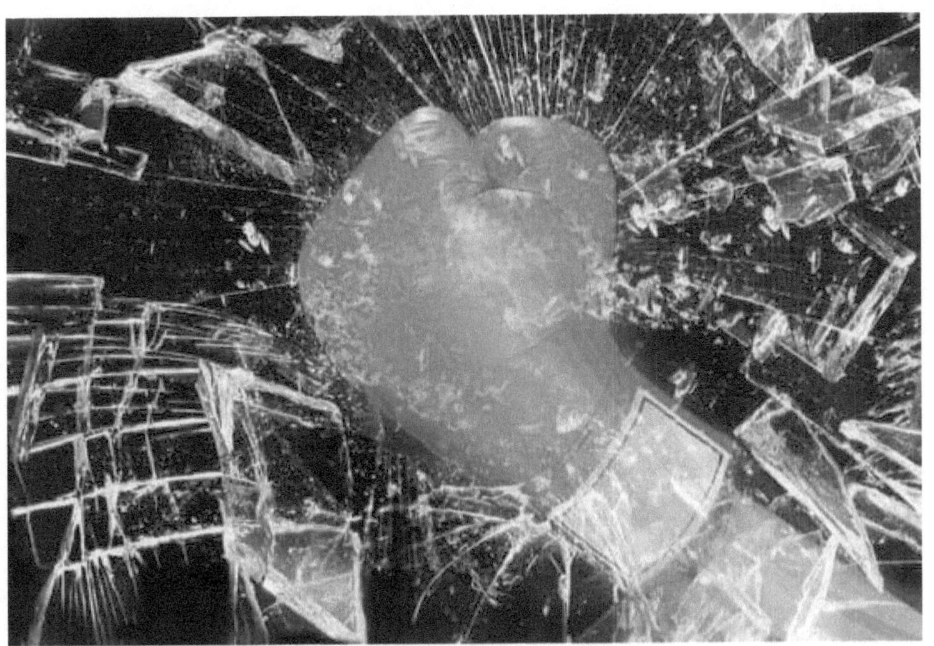

Chapter 5

Boost Metabolism and Loss Weight

Metabolism is commonly thought to be a matter of how fast or slowly you burn calories. We often hear people say, —I can't lose weight because I have a slow metabolism. In general, that is true, but metabolism is much more complex.

In this section, I'm going to give you few tips on the ways to improve your metabolic rate and take your weight loss to the next level. But before that, let's examine what Metabolism is and why is it important for you to have a high metabolic rate in order to lose weight.

Metabolism is the amount of energy (calories) your body burns to maintain itself. Whether you are eating, drinking, sleeping, cleaning etc.. your body is constantly burning calories to keep you going. Your metabolic rate is affected by your body composition. By body composition, I mean the total amount of muscle you have in your body against the total number of fat. Muscle used more calories to maintain itself than fat utilities. People who are more muscular (and have a lower percentage of body fat) are said to have a higher metabolism than others that are less muscular.

Here's how the metabolism works: Someone with a high metabolic rate is able to burn calories more efficiently than someone with a slower metabolic rate. Any calories that are not burned out get converted to fat. Let' s take a look at the three main types of calorie burn that happen throughout your day.

Calories burn #1: The majority of the calorie burn comes from your basal or resting Metabolism, which means you burn calories while you're doing absolutely nothing at all. Yes, 60 to 80 percent of your daily calories are burned up by just doing nothing. Whether it' s watching TV, sitting in a meeting at work, or sleeping, you are continuing to burn calories. The reason is that your body is always in a constant state of motion. Your heart is beating, blood is pumping through your veins, and your lungs are breathing.

Exercise is important for cardio health, but the calories you burn from exercise don't account for the majority of caloric burn happening throughout the day while doing absolutely nothing (your basal metabolism). The calories you burn during your one hour at the gym are relatively insignificant compared to all the calories you burn during the other twenty-three hours in the day. It's more productive to focus on naturally increasing the rate of your resting Metabolism—i.e., your caloric burn throughout the day.

Calories burn #2: The effect of simply eating and digesting your food accounts for about 10 to 15 percent of the calories you burn each day. Studies have shown that during the eating process, your metabolism increases by as much as 30 percent, and this effect lasts up to three hours after you have finished eating. How much caloric burn occurs depends on the type of food you eat.

More caloric burn is used to digest protein (25 calories burned for every 100 calories consumed) than to digest fats and carbohydrates (about 10 to 15 calories burned for every 100 calories consumed).

Calories burn #3: About 10 to 15 percent of your calorie burn comes from increasing your heart rate, strengthening your muscles, or physical activity, even light physical activity such as walking up the stairs.

How to Avoid Slowing Your Metabolism

One of the greatest myths about weight loss is that for some people, it is harder to lose weight because they have a genetically slow metabolism. However, scientific research shows that this is simply not true. Your metabolic rate is not fixed for life, and, in fact, it can and be re-fixed.

Here are seven ways to boost your metabolism to burn more calories:

1. Eat breakfast.

Have a hearty breakfast to rev up your metabolism for the day. Eating a high-protein breakfast wakes up your liver and kicks your metabolism into gear. A high- protein breakfast can increase your metabolic rate by 30 percent for up to twelve hours, which is the calorie-burning equivalent of a three- to five-mile jog. It is crucial to feed your body every three to four hours and not skip any meals. You especially don't want to skip breakfast. When you skip breakfast, it means your body goes without fuel for about fifteen hours including the overnight hours. This causes it to automatically store fat over the next twenty-four hours because it thinks it's in starvation mode or a deprived state.

2. Eat more frequently.

The goal is to not let more than four hours passes without a meal or snack. Yes, ironically, it is important to eat to lose weight! The number of times you eat is important to keep your metabolism revved up. Every time you eat, you have to burn calories in order to digest your food and eating increases your metabolic rate. When more than five hours pass without eating, your body automatically lowers its metabolic rate. In contrast, by eating meals and snacks throughout the day, your body stays at a steady metabolic burn rate that helps you burn calories and fat all day. Remember we are eating every three or four hours because eating less will slow your metabolism. It sends a signal to your body that it is starving and deprived, causing the body to respond by slowing the metabolic rate and holding on to existing fat reserves in the body. So, eat more. Yes, you can do that!

3. Drink more cold water.

German researchers found that if you drink six cups of cold water a day, it can raise resting metabolism by about 50 calories daily, which in a year can help you to shed about five pounds. This is because it takes more work for the body to heat the water to your body temperature. small thing that can help you lose weight with very little effort. The Germany researchers also suggest that for up to 90 minutes after drinking cold water, you will keep your metabolism boosted by as much as 24 percent over your average metabolism rate.

4. Don't eat right before going to bed.

Eating before bed is a guaranteed way to slow your metabolism and gain weight. The easy solution is to eat dinner and give yourself at least two to three hours after you eat before you go to sleep. You may even want to eat more lightly at dinner and the heaviest at breakfast. Getting more of your energy from your food earlier in the day helps you lose and maintain weight loss because your body can burn fat throughout the entire day. The fat-burning systems in the body slow, rest and repair at night while you're sleeping.

5. Drink caffeinated coffee or tea.

Caffeine is a central nervous system stimulant and can speed up your metabolism by 5 to 8 percent, which helps to burn about 100 to 175 calories a day. This does not mean you should overdo it and drink several cups of coffee. Having one cup of coffee is sufficient, but too many cups of coffee can have adverse side effects. Additionally, green tea, my favorite metabolism booster, is found to provide many health benefits to the body.

6. Get moving.

Physical activity of any kind speeds up metabolism, and aerobic exercise gives it a significant boost. Also, the higher the intensity of the aerobic exercise, the more it will help your metabolism remain elevated for an extended period of time, so that you continue to burn calories even after you have stopped exercising.

7. Spice it up.

One study showed that hot or spicy peppers (chili or cayenne peppers) caused a temporary metabolism boost of about 23 percent. Some people have even purchased cayenne pepper capsules to supplement spicy pepper into their diet daily just to boost their metabolism.

Once you begin to boost your metabolism, the body weight reduced and stay off permanently. Not only that, but your health will improve as well. You can learn how to speed up your metabolism so you burn more calories and fat throughout each day.

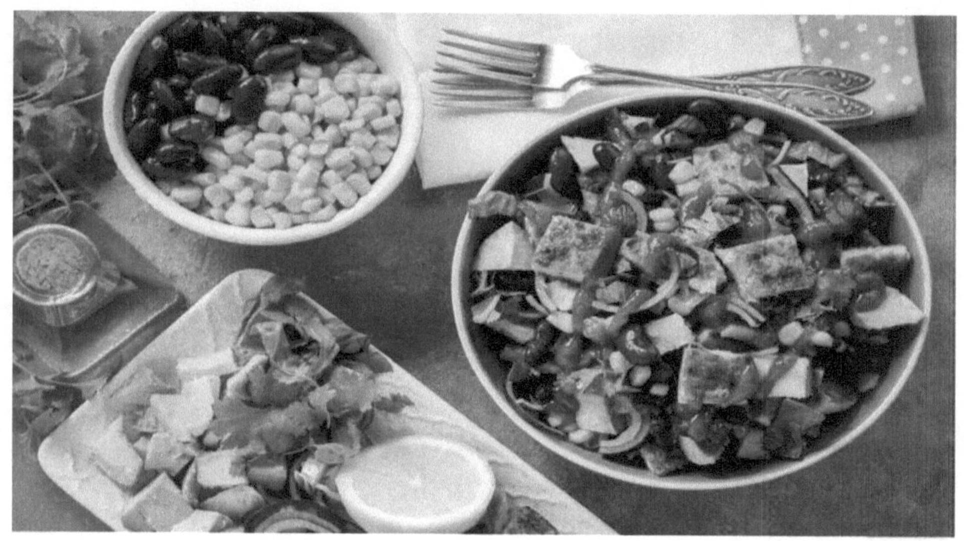

14 DAYS BOOST UP METABOLISM DIET PLAN

Natural Method to Boost body Metabolism

This **14 Days Programs** will be introducing some dairy product and some meat Protein to promote better fat burning. At the same time follow the below table for the intake of Macha pills and Rice Vinegar to accompany with the High Protein diet to further Boost Metabolism Program.

Japanese Rice Vinegar is mild in taste and more palatable to consume and wash down with warm water.

Rice Vinegar benefits are, improve Fatigue, is Liver Tonic, Improve Gut Health and Immunity, promote Radiant Skin and keep weight in check etc.

Consume After each Meal.

Weight size	Per day	Matcha	Japanese Rice Vinegar (tbsp)
50 -80 kgs	Breakfast	2	1
	Lunch	2	1
	Dinner		
90 - 120kgs	Breakfast	3	2
	Lunch	3	2
	Dinner		
130 - 160kgs	Breakfast	4	3
	Lunch	4	3
	Dinner		

If your body over-reactive to high doses, try to reduce the amount of intake and continue to monitor your system. If discomfort persists stop immediately.

For best result, by reducing the intake of a minimum of 500 Calories per day will see the result by the end of 14 days.

To measure your Calories by finding out your current weight size, an example of

Female weigh   80 kgs x 2 x 11 = 1760 – 500 = 1260 Calories

in-take per day

Male weigh   160 kgs x 2 x 12 = 2880 – 500 = 2380 Calories

in-take per day

You can refer to the Food Facts Table Guide at the end of this chapter to plan your meal according.

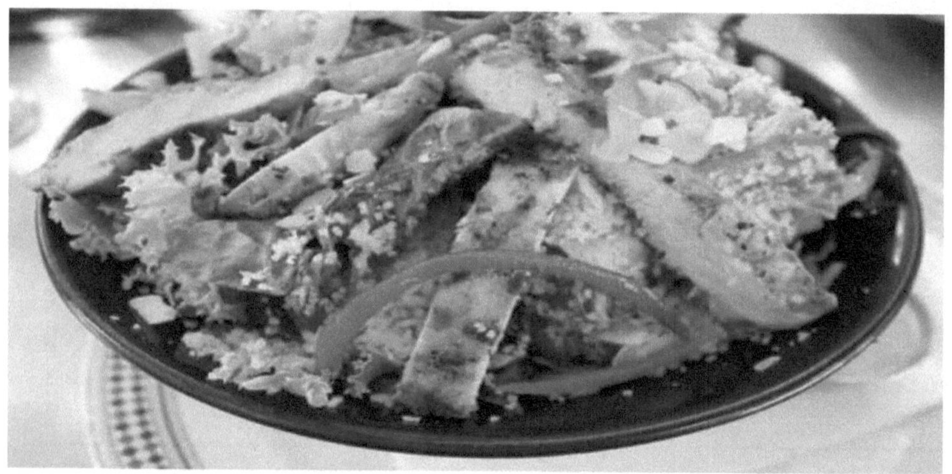

High Protein, Low Fat & Low Carbo Recipes

Chicken Breast is one of the great sources of protein with low fat and 0 Carbohydrate and is easy to prepare.

There are many tasty cooking methods for Chicken Breast too.

Food Item	Quantity	Calories	Pro (g)	Carbs (g)	Fat (g)
chicken breast	3 oz	143	26.5	0	3.8

#Tips

Prepare a batch of meat for one week to easy cooking process.

Clean the meat with salt bath, slice into strips of approximate 5 x 2 inches.

Lightly marinate with Pink salt, Black peppr, Cayenne Pepper Powder, grated ginger, store in freezer to ensure freshness.

Ready for Grill, Baked, Pan-Fried, Stir fried etc.

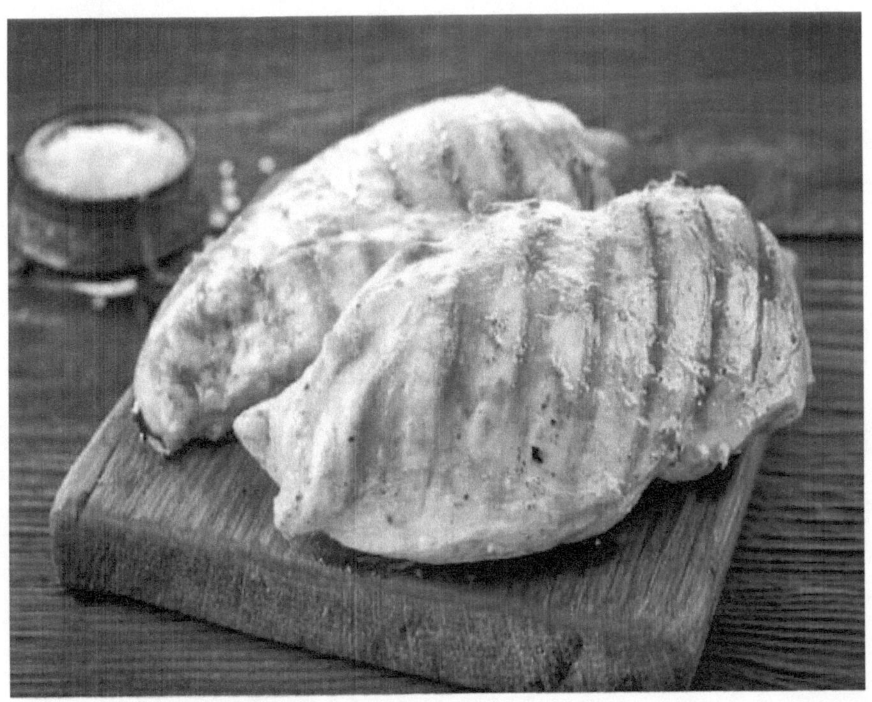

Baked Chicken with Melt Cheese

Serving : 1

Preparation time : 5 minutes

Cooking time: 8 minutes

Total : Calories 161.3g Protein 21.5g

Chicken Breast 2oz/170g   *(Calories 95.3g, Protein 18g)*

Mozzarella cheese 42g   *(Calories 36g. Protein 3.5g)*

1 teaspoon of Butter   *(Calories 30, Protein 0g)*

Turn on the Oven to 200 deg C setting, Time 8 minutes.

Baking Tray lightly oil, rub the olive oil on the meat, lay the meat nicely on the trap and top with cheese and grill

Top with some Coriander / Parsley, squeeze some lime juice, combine this dish with either grill vegetable (egg plants, zucchini, capsicum), Boil Veggie or beans or Pan-fried potatoes or Green salad.

Baked Honey Chicken with Balsamic reduction vinegar

Serving : 1

Preparation time : 5 minutes

Cooking time: 8 minutes

Total : Calories 155.3g Protein 18g

Chicken Breast 2oz/170g   (Calories 95.3g, Protein 18g)

1 teaspoon Raw Honey   (Calories 20g. Protein 0g)

1 teaspoon of Olive oil   (Calories 40g. Protein 0g)

1 teaspoon of minced garlic

Rub all the ingredients on the meat, let it marinate for 1 hours.

Turn on the Oven to 200 deg C setting, Time 8 minutes.

Baking Tray lightly oil, lay the meat nicely on the trap.

Top with Balsamic reduction vinegar, combine this dish with Grill Veggie & cooked Edamame.

Grill Masala Chicken

Serving : 1

Preparation time : 10 minutes

Cooking time: 8 minutes

Total : Calories 210.3g Protein 21g

Chicken Breast 2oz/170g   (Calories 95.3g, Protein 18g)

1 tablespoon Plain Yogurt   (Calories 25g. Protein 0.5g)

1 teaspoon of Butter   (Calories 30g. Protein 0g)

1 teaspoon of minced garlic

2 teaspoons of Masala or curry power   (Calories 50g. Protein 1.8g)

1 teaspoon of lime juice

A pinch of cumin seed *optional

Rub all the ingredients on the meat, let it marinate for 2 hours or more.

Turn on the Oven to 200 deg C setting, Time 8 minutes.

Baking Tray lightly oil, lay the meat nicely on the trap.

Top with some Coriander / Parsley, squeeze some lime juice, combine this dish with Grill potatoes and Green salad.

Skinny Hot Chocolate Drink

Serving : 1

Preparation time : 5 minutes

Cooking time: 5 minutes

Total : Calories 190.2g Protein 9.2g

1 tablespoon of Hershey Baking Cocoa   (Calories 34.2g, Protein 0.2)

Half tablespoon of Hershey semi-sweet chocolate   (Calories 70, Protein 1)

1 cup Skim Milk   (Calories 86, Protein 8)

1/4 teaspoon of vanilla extract

Simmer Milk in a pot with the chocolate till the chocolate melted, put 2 tablespoon of liquid to the cocoa powder stir till well dissolved and add in the rest of liquid.

Great Energy Booster Drink!

Egg White is a great way to Protein to enhance metabolism rate with 0 Fat and low in Carbohydrates.

Food Item	Quantity	Calories	Pro (g)	Carbs (g)	Fat (g)
egg whites	4	68	14	1.8	0
egg, whole	1	75	6.3	0.6	5

Oatmeal Porridge

Serving : 1

Preparation time : 5 minutes

Cooking time: 8 minutes

Total : Calories 209g Protein 12.5g

3 tablespoon of Raw Oats   (Calories 114g, Protein 4)

2 tablespoon of Sweet Corn   (Calories 35, Protein 1)

1 Egg White   (Calories 17, Protein 3.5)

1/2 cup Skim Milk   (Calories 43, Protein 4)

Pinch of Pink salt to taste

Simmer Milk in a pot with Raw Oats cook for 3 minutes, pour in the sweet corn and stir in the egg white in low fire, remove pot once the egg white turn white and add a pinch of salt to taste.

Poached Egg Bento set

Serving : 1

Preparation time : 15 minutes

Cooking time:10 minutes

Total : Calories 153.5g Protein 18.9g

Chicken Breast 1oz/85g	*(Calories 48g, Protein 9g)*
1 teaspoon of Butter	*(Calories 30g. Protein 0g)*
2 Poached Egg White	(Calories 34g, Protein 7g)
2 tablespoons of Boiled Edamame	(Calories 24g, Protein 2g)
1/2 cup of Chopped Cucumber	(Calories 8g, Protein 0.3g)
2 tablespoon of Toasted Nori (seaweed)	(Calories 4g, Protein 0.6g)
1 tablespoon of Kimchi (Optional)	(Calories 5.5g, Protein 0g)

Pan fried the Chicken breast with butter. Slice into bite size.

Boil a small pot of water with 1/2 teaspoon of rice vinegar, add the Egg white once water is in boiling temperature.

Placed Egg at the center of a large plate and all the ingredient at the side of the plate.

***The Egg white is a rice replacement.**

Edamame Hummus

Serving : 10

Preparation time : 30 minutes

Cooking time: 10 minutes

Total : Calories 1288.4g Protein 64.21g

Per serving Calories 130g Protein 6.4g

(A) 500g of Boiled Edamame   (Calories 610g, Protein 55g)

 2 tablespoons of chopped Garlic   (Calories 8.4g, Protein 0.4g)

 1/2 cup of Lime Juice   (Calories 26g, Protein 0.31g)

 3 tablespoon of Olive oil   (Calories 360g, Protein 0g)

(B) 50g of Toasted Sesame seeds   (Calories 284g, Protein 8.5g)

 10g of Toasted Cumin seeds

 Pink salt to taste

Blend (A) ingredient with 1/4 cup of ice-cold water until is smooth and creamy.

Grind (B) till powder texture. Add into (A) with salt to taste.

Store Hummus in a few small containers in the freeze to keep fresh and longer shelf live. Is a great healthy snack with Cucumber, Carrots, & Capsicum sticks.

Adhered to this Detox Program with these Green Food Diet for 14 Days to enjoy a significant result.

#Note: All the Calories & Protein provided may be varied is only serve as a guideline.

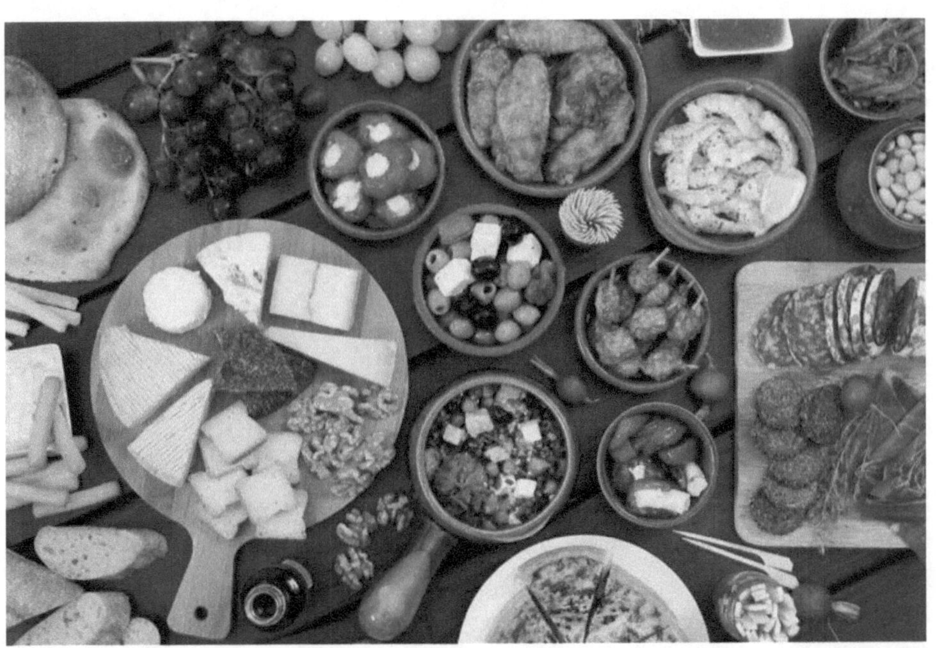

Food Source Calories & Protein Table

Meat, Poultry, Eggs:

Food (Cooked)Serving	Size	Calories	Protein (g)
Chicken, skinless	85 g	141	28
Steak	85 g	158	26
Turkey, roasted	85 g	135	25
Lamb	85 g	172	23
Pork	85 g	122	22
Ham	85 g	139	14
Egg, large	1 egg	71	16

Seafood:

Food (Cooked)Serving	Size (3oz)	Calories	Protein(g)
Salmon	85 g	155	22
Tuna	85 g	99	22
Shrimp	85 g	101	20
Lobster	85 g	76	16

Legumes, Grains:

Name of Food (Cooked)	Size (cup)	Calories	Protein (g)
Pinto Beans	½	197	11
Adzuki Beans	½	147	9
Lentils	½	101	9
Edamame	½	95	9
Black Beans	½	114	8
Red Kidney Beans	½	112	8
Chickpeas	½	134	7
Black-eyed Peas	½	100	7
Fava Beans	½	94	7
Lima Beans	½	105	6
Quinoa	½	111	4
Peas, Green	½	59	4

Nuts and Seeds:	Size	Calories	Protein (g)
Soy Nuts	1oz	120	12
Pumpkin Seeds	1oz	159	9
Peanuts	1oz	166	7
Peanut Butter	1 Tbsp	188	7
Almonds	1oz	163	6
Pistachios	1oz	161	6
Flax Seeds	1oz	140	6
Sunflower Seeds	1oz	140	6
ChiaSeeds	1oz	138	5
Walnuts	1oz	185	4
Cashews	1oz	162	4

DairyProducts:	Size	Calories	Protein (g)
Greek Yogurt	6 oz	100	18
Cottage Cheese (1% fat)	4 oz	81	14
Regular Yogurt (nonfat)	225g	100	11
Milk, Skim	1 cup	86	8
Soy milk	1 cup	132	8
Mozzarella (part skim)	1 oz	72	7
String Cheese (nonfat)	0.75 oz	50	6
Cheddar Cheese	1 oz	114	7
Coconut Yogurt	2/3 cup	150	13

FRUITS Products:	Size	Calories	Protein (g)
Banana	½ cup	69	0.8
Watermelon	½ cup	24.3	0.5
Apricot	½ cup	39.6	1.2
Strawberry	½ cup	25	0.5
Cantalope	½ cup	27.3	0.7
Apple	½ cup	36.9	0.1
Orange	½ cup	42.3	0.8

Vegetables:

Name of Food	Size (cup)½	Calories	Protein (g)
Spinach, cooked		20.7	2.7
Cucumber		6.8	0.4
Egg Plant, cooked		13.9	0.4
Cabbage		11.1	0.6
Broccoli, cooked		21.8	2.3
Cauliflower		14.3	1.1
Carrot, cooked		35	0.9
Tomatoes		18.9	0.8
Bell Peppers		19	0.8
Onion		30.4	0.9
Sweet Potatoes, cooked		103	1.7
Potatoes		83	1.46
Romaine Lettuces *ONE CUP		7.8	1
Celery, cooked		13.5	0.6
Pumpkin, cooked		24.5	0.9
Mushroom		21.1	1.7
Zucchini, cooked		14.4	0.5

Chapter 6

Motivate Yourself to Exercise

Exercise is one of the major factors in any weight loss program. But knowing how much exercise you need, when to start, and what type of exercise is suitable for you can be a little confusing, especially if you are a beginner. There are exercise programs that include strength training, flexibility, cardio, and a combination of two or more of them.

So what kind of exercise and how much of it do you need to lose weight? Experts say that the best training to lose weight is simply any kind of exercise that you will do: this means going out and taking a walk every day on a regular basis. Over time your walks will become easier and you'll want to increase the distance. You'll notice a difference in how you feel quickly once you get up and start moving.

Oftentimes people stop doing exercises out of boredom or because they'll get or aggravate some kind of injury. It is recommended that you engage in exercises that you can easily do in the beginning like walking or biking. As you progress you can begin doing more strenuous exercise but give your body a chance to adapt to physical activity again first. Injuries can be a major setback, especially if you're older. It's okay to push yourself a little as you progress but listen to your body when it's telling you it's hurting and back off.

Below are several tips that will help you stick to a weight loss workout program:

Exercise with a friend or try to have an exercise partner during your workouts.

Try to make a schedule or calendar for your workouts.

Weighing yourself regularly at the same time every week can help you keep on track to reach your weight loss goal.

Avoid getting over-motivated by doing too much and too fast.

Cook your own meals instead of eating out to control the amount of calories you consume.

Cut back on drinking wine, beer, or any alcoholic beverages.

On the other hand, if you are not in a good physical condition to do any weight loss exercises, **the following are some guidelines that will help you get the best results eventually:**

Try to start slowly and gradually with your chosen weight loss exercise.

You can simply start walking for 10 minutes per day for a couple weeks. This will get you up and moving and in the habit of doing it. After that start increasing your time by five minutes every two weeks. Within a couple of months you'll be walking 30 minutes per day.

Engage in the right exercises.

Do regular aerobic exercises, but do them in short bursts of 10-20 minute sessions.

Understand that the effect of exercises on your body is cumulative, meaning that you can only see significant changes after a few weeks or more.

Retain your water supply. In other words, drink plenty of water, not soda, tea, juice, sports drinks, etc. Simple h20 is the best thing for your body.

By exercising regularly, the body fat is used more as fuel for physical activities, thus reserving the body's carbohydrates for emergency situations and more strenuous activities.

No matter what type of exercises you choose for losing weight, if you do it regularly with patience, you can be sure you are on the right track.

Some of the best exercises that are proven to burn most calories are:

Step Aerobics - Aerobics is often included in most exercise programs to lose weight. Done correctly, you will see results in a matter of two weeks!

Brisk Walking - a very easy cardio workout that you can fit in your daily activities. It also helps tone your legs, hips, and stomach.

Jogging/Running - very good for your body and helps burn a lot of calories without even going to the gym.

Hiking - should not be confused with leisurely walk. Hiking can burn around 350 calories an hour.

Yoga - a relaxing way to lose weight by involving stretching and improves the body's flexibility too. There are more advanced and difficult moves which you can combine for other positions.

Bicycling - aside from being enjoyable, this exercise is a great way to burn calories. You can also invest in an exercise bike if you don't have much available time to go out riding.

Swimming - certainly one of the best exercise to lose weight and also tones your entire body.

Dancing - another fun and excellent weight loss exercise and tones the entire body.

Body Weight Training - should be a part of any weight loss exercise program which you can do for an hour or 30 minutes a day, three times a week. Avoid lifting weights! This can lead to injury. Your body weight is sufficient for what you want to accomplish.

Exercise CDs/DVDs - you can find a lot of these CDs/DVDs to help you tone up and lose weight. Choose a high energy and aim to do it once a day regularly.

Horseback Riding - doing this once a week can help you stay fit while enjoying the nature around you during your ride.

Zumba - can burn a lot of calories in just one hour.

Soccer - a sporty way to burn calories by running around the soccer field.

Gardening - tending to the garden - cleaning, pulling out weeds, planting - can also be a way to burn calories.

House Cleaning - tidying up your home and multi-tasking in different household chores can also burn a lot of calories.

Proper exercise and a healthy diet are effective in any weight loss programs. People often make the mistake that they can eat whatever they want since they do a lot of exercises. Remember, not eating the unwanted calories is far easier than burning them off in the future. Keep in mind also that keeping the weight off once you've lost it is what makes any weight loss program successful.

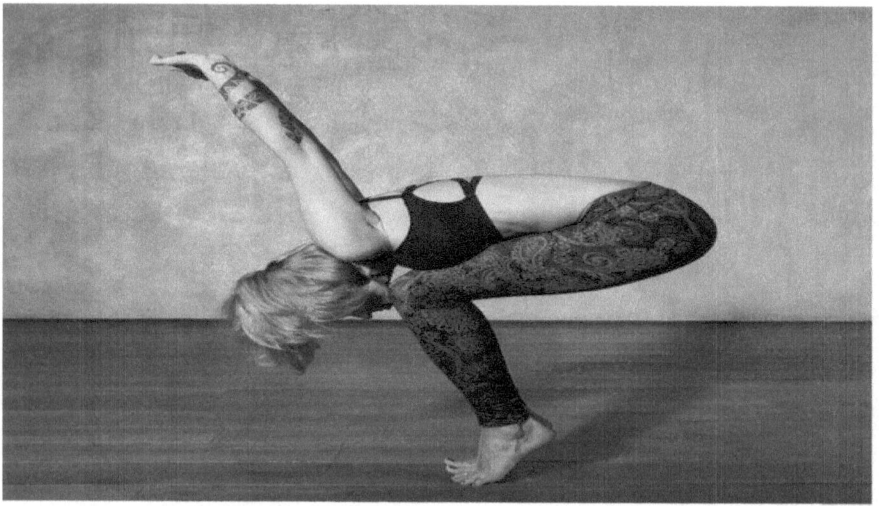

Chapter 7

28 Days Action Plan Program

Welcome to this chapter, use the following journal to track your progress on weight lose and implement menus later in this chapter to achieve your goals

I encourage you to begin with a baby step and gradually increase the momentum.

DAY 0

Invest on a **FITNESS Watch** to help you to keep track and monitor on your step counts, calories burn, sleeping pattern on each day. **Get committed with at least 10,000 step a day by the end of this 30 days program.** Get your Pink Healthy back.

Create a Vision Board – Pin your desire figure/ model you aim to achieved.

Take a Selfie and weight to place next to your idea weight model picture.

Start a Journal for Weight Management. Be honest with yourself, write

down how the weight you intent to loss in 10 days. What diet you need to

stay away and be strong to stay in the program – **STAY COMMITED!**

DAY 1 to 7

Begin your DETOX & GREEN FOOD Diet Program

Half hour - Exercise Program each day

Record your daily activities and results

End of the day go through your Journal on the area you need to improve

and adjust.

*Dinner (ensure the last intake before 8 pm)

DAY 8 to14

DETOX & GREEN FOOD Diet Program

Forty-Five minutes - Exercise Program each day

Record your daily activities and results

End of the day, go through your Journal on the area you need to improve and adjust.

*Dinner (ensure the last intake before 8 pm)

DAY 15, 16 (Rejoice day)

Take a break from your Diet Program.

Reward yourself for what you had achieved, by now you should be down with at least ONE Kilogram or more. Congratulations!

Forty-Five minutes - Exercise Program each day

Record your daily activities and results

End of the day go through your Journal on the area you need to improve and adjust.

*Dinner (ensure the last intake before 8 pm)

DAY 17 – 30 days (total duration 14 Days)

Begin your High Protein Metabolism Booster Diet Program

ONE Hour - Exercise Program each day

Record your daily activities and results

End of the day go through your Journal on the area you need to improve and adjust. *(Dinner (ensure the last intake before 8 pm)

Tracking of Progress

To better my health, my goal is to lose _______ pounds. I will accomplish this through:

Physical activity (list exercise plans):

Eating more low-calorie, nutritious foods like:

Changing the following eating habits:

WEEK 1	DATE	WEIGHT	Remarks	
Day 1			Progress!	It's too early to tell!
Day 2			Progress!	It's too early to tell!
Day 3			Progress!	It's too early to tell!
Day 4			No weight loss yet	It's too early to tell!
Day 5			Doing well	I'll try harder
Day 6			Doing well	I'll try harder
Day 7			I lost a little weight!	I'll try harder

WEEK 2	DATE	WEIGHT	Remarks (pick from bottom of page or write your own)
Day 8			
Day 9			
Day 10			
Day 11			
Day 12			
Day 13			
Day 14			

WEEK 3	DATE	WEIGHT	Remarks
Day 15			
Day 16			
Day 17			
Day 18			
Day 19			
Day 20			
Day 21			

WEEK 4	DATE	WEIGHT	Remarks
Day 22			
Day 23			
Day 24			
Day 25			
Day 26			
Day 27			
Day 28			

WEEK 5	DATE	WEIGHT	Remarks
Day 29			
Day 30			

Positive Remarks: I'm doing pretty well. Feeling good. Exercise isn't so bad. Great job!

Other remarks: I need to try harder. Bummer. No change this week – oh well.

1600 Calories Baseline – 500 = 1100 Calories Per Day Meal Plan

DAY ONE PLAN	Food Item			Quantity	Calories(g)	Protein (g)
Breakfast	Chocolate drink 190.2 Calories, 9.2 Protein	Chia seed Parfait 363 Calories, 18.5 Protein		1 serving	553.2	27.7
Tea Break	Banana			1/2 cup	69	0.8
Lunch	Masala Chicken 210.3 Calories, 21Protein	Boil Broccoli 21.8 Calories, 2.3 Protein		1 serving	232.1	23.3
Tea Break	Cantelope 27.3 Calories, 0.7Protein	cheese stick 50 calories, 6 Protein		1/2 cup	77.3	6.7
Dinner	Avocado Taco			1 serving	190	9.5
				Meal #1 Subtotals:	1121.6	68

DAY TWO PLAN	Food Item			Quantity	Calories(g)	Protein (g)
Breakfast	Egg Bento set 153.5 Calories, 18.9 Protein			2 serving	307	37.8
Tea Break	Coconut Yogurt 150 Calories, 13 Protein	Apple 36.9 Calories, 0.1 Protein		1/2 cup	186.9	13.1
Lunch	Soba Combo 215 Calories, 63.5 Protein				215	63.5
Tea Break	Steam sweet Potatoes 103 Calories, 1.7 Protein	Almond 40 g 80 Calories, 3 Protein		1/2 cup	183	3.7
Dinner	Honey Chicken 155.3 Calories, 18 Protein	Boil Spinach 41 Calories, 3 Protein	Tomatoes 18.9 Calories, 0.8 Protein	1 serving & 1/2 cup	215.2	21.8
				Meal #2 Subtotals:	1107.1	139.9

2000 Calories Baseline – 500 = 1500 Calories Per Day Meal Plan

DAY ONE PLAN	Food Item		Quantity	Calories(g)	Protein (g)
Breakfast	Soba Combo 215 Calories, 63.5 Protein	Chia seed Parfait 363 Calories, 18.5 Protein	2 serving Of Soba + 1 serving Parfait	793	145.5
Tea Break	Banana		1/2 cup	69	0.8
Lunch	Masala Chicken 210.3 Calories, 21Protein	Boil Broccoli 21.8 Calories, 2.3 Protein	1 serving	232.1	23.3
Tea Break	Cantelope 27.3 Calories, 0.7Protein		1/2 cup	27.3	0.7
Dinner	Avocado Taco 190Calories, 9.5Protein	Chocolate drink 190.2 Calories, 9.2 Protein		380.2	18.7
			Meal #1 Subtotals:	1501.6	189

DAY TWO PLAN	Food Item			Quantity	Calories(g)	Protein (g)
Breakfast	Egg Bento set 153.5 Calories, 18.9 Protein			3 serving	460.5	56.7
Tea Break	Coconut Yogurt 150 Calories, 13 Protein	Apple 36.9 Calories, 0.1 Protein		1/2 cup	186.9	13.1
Lunch	Honey Chicken 155.3 Calories, 18 Protein	Boil Spinach 41 Calories, 3 Protein	Tomatoes 18.9 Calories, 0.8 Protein	2 serving & 1/2 cup	430.4	43.6
Tea Break	Almond			1 oz	163	6
Dinner	Waldof Salad				276	7.31
				Meal #2 Subtotals:	1516.8	126.71

Celebrate the NEW YOU

After these 30 Days Program, by now you should be weighing 2 – 3 kilograms less than before.

If this is not your targeted weight, you can continue these 30 programs after your Diet Break day. You are familiar with the cycle by monitoring and tracking all your movement. Re-access your journal and tracking table to fine-tune your program accordingly.

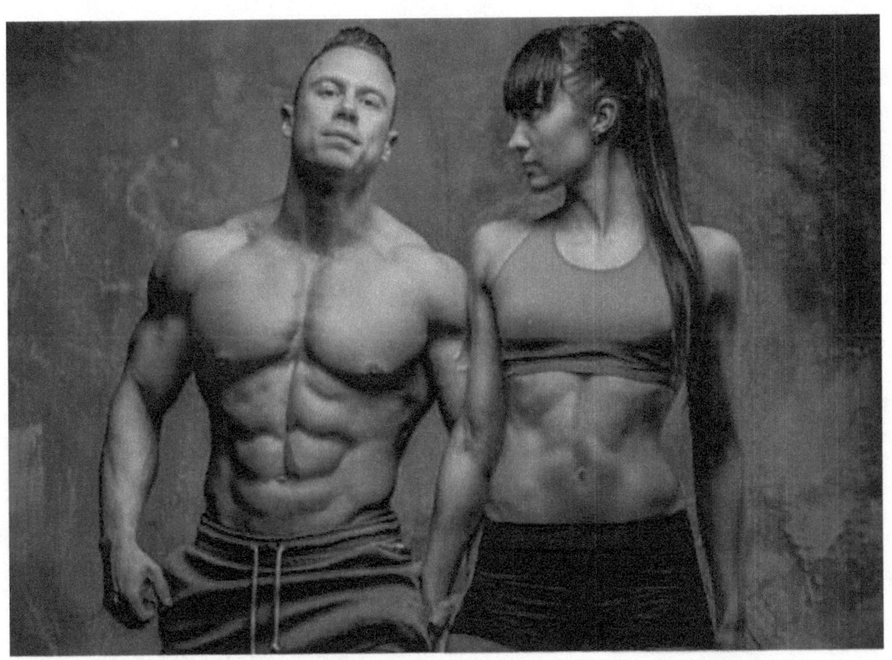

Chapter 8

Ten Healthy Ways to Lose Weight Fast

Have you ever walked down the street, into a restaurant, or practically anywhere public - and noticed that a large percentage people are either overweight or downright obese? Just 20 years ago, the opposite was true. Sadly, unless you're one of the minority who is lean and fit - this type of landscape can create a setting where you simply want to give up on your own weight loss goals.

That said, there's always hope if you're willing to keep an open mind and make a few changes. In this article, I'll share the top ten healthy ways to lose weight fast - whether you're following a diet or not!

Ten Healthy Ways to Lose Weight Fast!

1. Walk everyday!

Walking will help you set a positive intention. Plus you'll stay more motivated, by being connected to your environment. Try and reach 45 minutes each day, but even 10-15 minutes will help.

2. Add cayenne pepper and/or lemon to your water, and DRINK.

Cayenne pepper and lemon (or lime) are both known to stimulate the metabolism and encourage weight loss. By sipping about two liters of water per day, you'll keep your metabolism running high, while flushing out fats.

3. Cut your portions down a bit by using smaller dishes.

Trade out your dinner plates for a large salad plate, and you'll hardly notice your portions shrink. You can reduce your food intake at meals by 10-30% without hardly noticing.

Eat your Five Veggies each day!

Have Veggies at every snack and meal. I add peppers, onion and garlic to my eggs, and top it off with salsa, rather than adding cheese. Veggies are delicious for mid-morning snacks, have some celery and raw almond butter for good staying power.

1. Reduce your sugar intake, eating it only once a day.

Many of us consumes sugar throughout the day, without even realizing it. We have a little in our coffee, along with say, Raisin Bran for breakfast. Then for lunch will have a soda or energy drink, and so on. Plus, sugar is added to most of the prepared foods we eat - so just try and eat whole foods as much as possible, limiting sugar to no more than 50 grams a day.

2. Try a Three day juice detox!

If you really need a boost to get your weight loss started, simply borrow a juicer from a friend and drink veggie juice for three days. I guarantee you'll feel lighter by the end of it, plus you'll better appreciate the healthy, simple foods when you complete the fast. (It's a good idea to check with your doc before juicing or starting any weight loss plan.)

3. Spice up your life!

It's a proven fact. Unless you have a particular disorder, flavorful and spicy foods are good for most people. As long as it agrees with you, eat lots of peppers, onions, garlic, leeks, cayenne pepper, red pepper, jalepeno and more — statistics shows that spicy foods keep your metabolism running higher for up to 3 hours after eating.

4. Eat more often.

Athletes have been doing this for decades. Eat smaller meals or snacks, 5-6 times a day. This helps avoid massive insulin spikes, which put the body into fat storage mode.

5. Replace most breads with lentils or other beans.

Lentils and other beans are a slower carb, so they give your body the carbohydrates it wants, without the fat storage that traditional breads encourage. Plus, most bread has sugar added to it, anyway. Sprouted grain breads are a better choice, if you really want bread.

6. Eat healthy fats, and lean proteins.

Try and minimize drinking milk, and instead eat a little low-fat Greek yogurt, cottage cheese, fish, eggs and chicken cooked in olive, coconut or macadamia nut oil.

There you have it. Follow these steps for healthy ways to lose weight fast and you should see noticeable results within a few weeks. And remember, visualize your positive outcome, seeing yourself lean and happy - you'll be more successful this way, and enjoy the process, too. I wish you success in your weight loss goals!

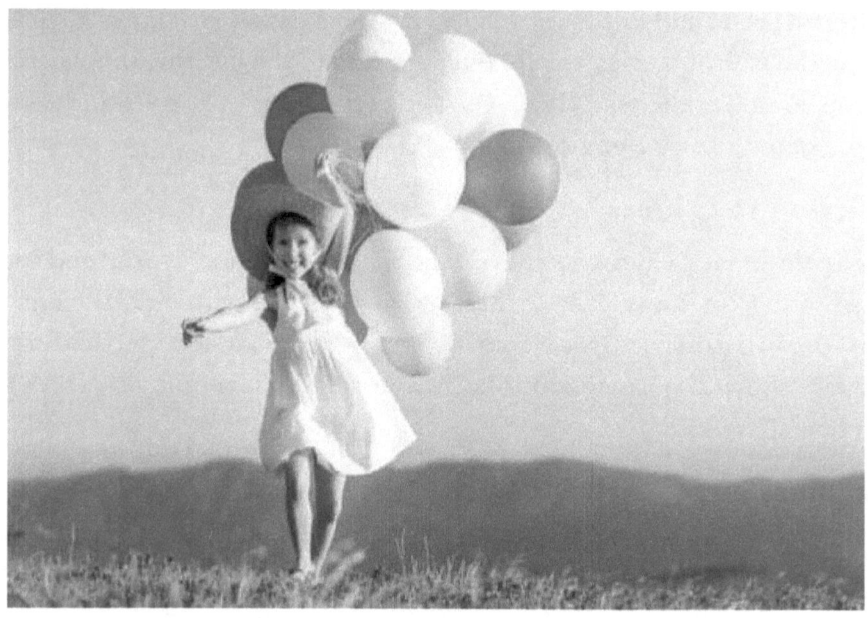

CONCLUSION

Remember that you have the power to change your life, and now with the information in this eBook, you have the tools to turn your dreams into reality. Everyday is a new beginning of the rest of your life. You are in control of what happens today. Start dreaming about your sexy, beautiful body and watch it become reality. You have the power over your body and your life, so live it with passion, because you only get one!

In closing, I wanted to leave you with my 8 Commandments for Looking Young and Feeling Great.

1. Thou shalt take responsibility for thine own health and well-being.

If you want to be healthy, have more energy, and feel great, you must take the time to learn what is involved and apply it to your own life. You have to watch what goes into your mouth, how much exercise or physical activity you get, and what thoughts you're thinking throughout the day.

2. Thou shalt sleep.

Sleep and rest is the body's way of recharging the system. Sleep is the easiest, yet most underrated activity for healing the body. Lack of sleep definitely saps your glow and instantly ages you, giving you puffy red eyes with dark circles under them.

3. Thou shalt detoxify and cleanse the body.

Detoxifying the body means is ridding the body of poisons and toxins so that you can speed up weight loss and restore great health. A clean body is a beautiful body!

4. Thou shalt eat healthier, natural, whole foods.

Healthy eating can turn back the hands of time and return the body to a more youthful state. When you eat natural foods, you simply look and feel better. You keep the body clean at the cellular level and look radiant despite your age. Eating healthy should be part of your —beauty regimen.

5. Thou shalt commit to a lifestyle change.

Losing weight permanently requires a commitment to change in your thinking, your lifestyle, your mindset. It requires gaining knowledge and making permanent changes in your life for the better!

6. Thou shalt embrace the journey.

This is a journey that will change your life; it's not a diet but a lifestyle! Be kind and supportive to yourself. Learn to applaud yourself for the smallest accomplishment. And when you slip up sometimes, know that it is okay; it is called being human.

7. Thou shalt live, love, and laugh.

Laughter is still good for the soul. Live your life with passion! Never give up on your dreams! And most importantly love! Remember that love never fails!

Now get your into gear and start working!

Sidney Griffith

http://www.Amazon.com/gp/customer-reviews/write-a-review.html?asin=B07XNYYZDT